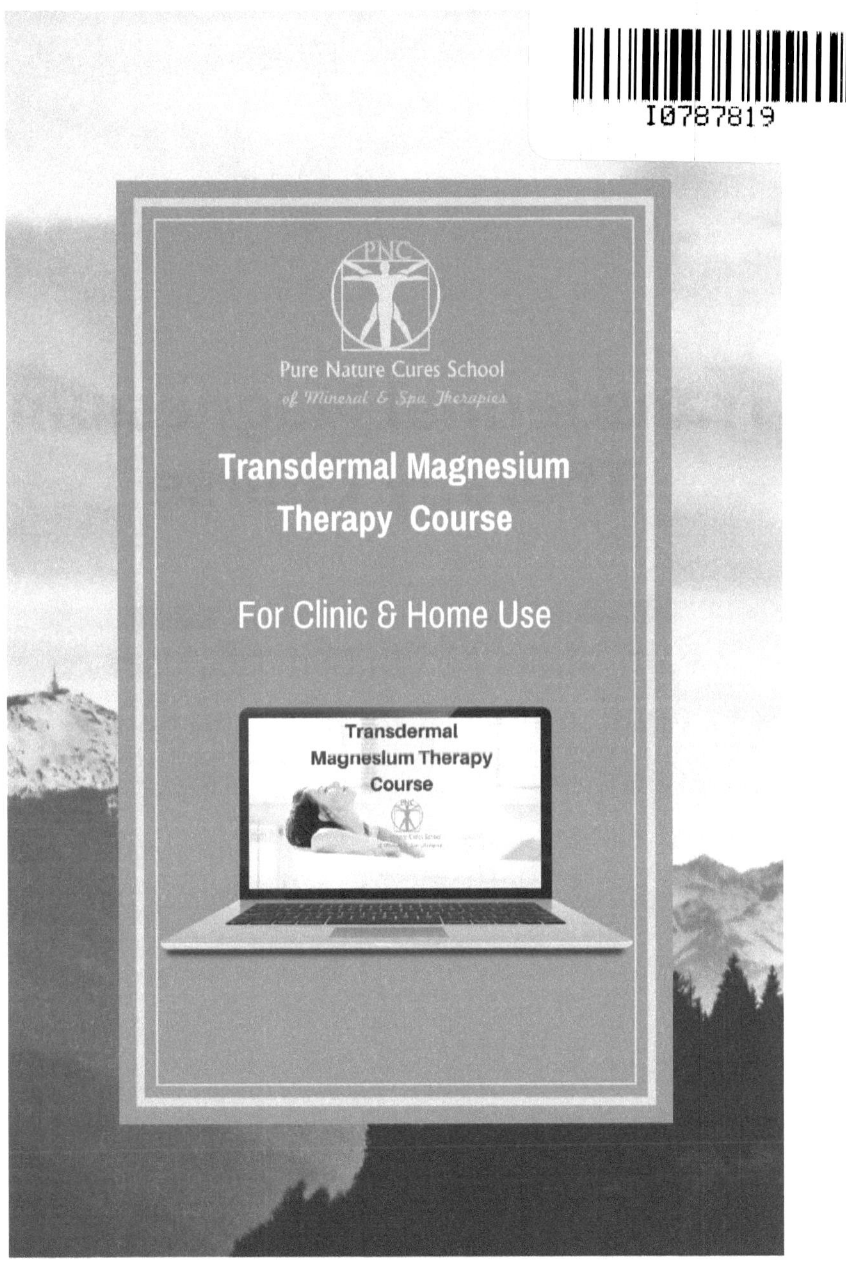
PNC
Pure Nature Cures School
of Mineral & Spa Therapies
Transdermal Magnesium
Therapy Course
For Clinic & Home Use
Transdermal
Magnesium Therapy
Course

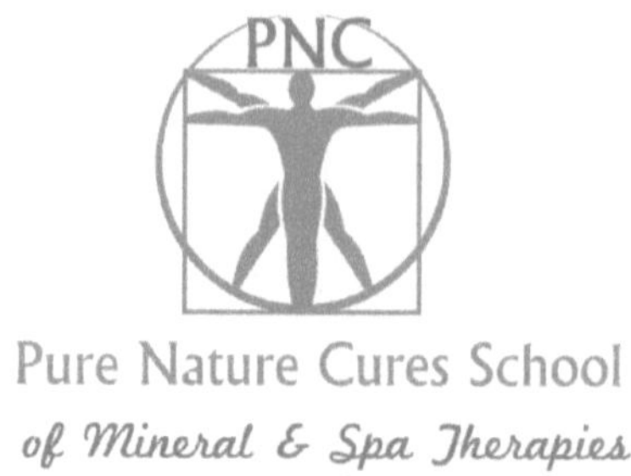

Transdermal Magnesium Therapy Course

Learn about health benefits, uses & applications of magnesium salts

Galina St George

Transdermal Magnesium Therapy Course for Clinic & Home Use

Transdermal Magnesium Therapy Course for Clinic & Home Use

Table of Contents

Introduction

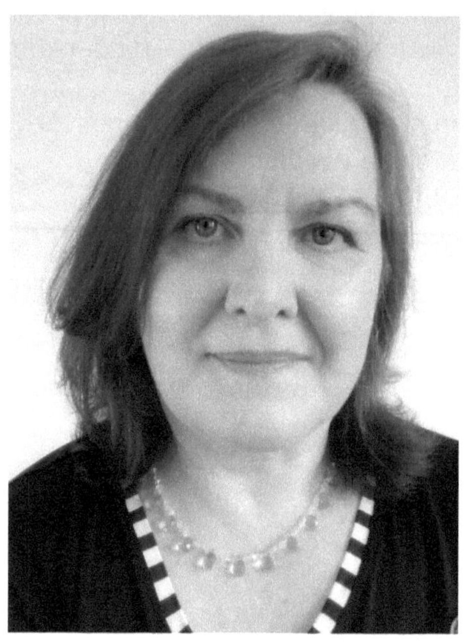

Magnesium is rightly called "the miracle mineral". There are few minerals which attract so much attention and instigate so much scientific research. The reason is that it not only participates in over 300 biochemical reactions in the body but helps maintain so many bodily functions, such as the normal muscle and nerve function, steady heart rhythm, normal blood pressure, healthy immune system and strong bones. It also helps maintain the blood sugar at normal levels. It plays a vital role in preventing heart disease, diabetes, cancer, osteoporosis and a whole range of other dangerous and debilitating diseases.

Magnesium deficiency is more common than we realise. It can be explained by many factors, with the main reasons being depletion of soil in minerals worldwide due to intensive agriculture. Another factor is a compromised digestive tract which includes a large number of people - young and old.

According to American nutritionists, an average adult needs 200mg more magnesium per day than what is obtained from a diet. The fact is that the dietary magnesium is not sufficient in providing the body with this important mineral.

Dr Carolyn Dean lists the following conditions which develop in cases of magnesium deficiency or and require magnesium supplementation:

"Acid reflux, Adrenal fatigue, Alzheimer's disease, Angina, Anxiety and panic attacks, Arthritis, Asthma,

Atherosclerosis, Blood clots, Bowel disease, Brain dysfunction, Bruxism or teeth grinding, Cholesterol elevation, cystitis, Depression, Detoxification, Diabetes, Fatigue, Headaches, Heart disease, Hypertension, Hypoglycemia, Indigestion, Inflammation, Insomnia, IBS, Kidney disease, Kidney stones, Migraine, Musculo-skeletal conditions: (muscle cramps, fibrositis, fibromyalgia, GI spasms, tension headaches, muscle spams or muscle contractions in any muscle of the body, chronic neck and back pain, jaw tension), Nerve problems – Neuralgia, Neuritis, Neuropathy (burning pain, muscle weakness, numbness paralysis, pins and needles, seizures and convulsions, tingling twitching, vertigo, confusion), Obstetrical and gynaecological problems (PMS, dysmenorrhea, female infertility, premature contractions, preeclampsia and eclampsia, cerebral palsy, sudden infant death syndrome, male infertility), Osteoporosis, Parkinson's disease, Raynaud's syndrome, Sports injuries, Sports recovery, Tongue biting, Tooth decay."
http://drcarolyndean.com.

While there are many excellent magnesium supplements on

the market, oral supplementation is not always effective due to our body inefficiency in absorbing it through the digestive tract. One of the reasons is that our intestinal tract gets covered by mucus as we grow older, or for other reasons. This means that we need to find other ways to bring sufficient magnesium to the body regularly. There is a fast way of doing it - through intravenous injections, but it's not an option for most people since it needs a professional to do it.

However, there is another, quick and simple method, to supplement this very important mineral. This method involves applying magnesium salts through the skin. The reason it is a hugely effective method is that our skin can absorb, so ions of magnesium penetrate through the skin into the bloodstream and get delivered to the cells needing it.

This course gives a very detailed explanation of various aspects of magnesium, its role in health, symptoms and consequences of magnesium deficiency for health and ways to supplement it through the skin. The course is created for therapists and members of the public wishing to learn it for their use. However, if you want to learn it in more detail or for professional use with an option to get certified, we can offer an online version of the course. You will be able to find information in the book. Alternatively, feel free to contact me for more details or if you have any questions.

Galina St George

Disclaimer

The author of this material sincerely believes that a natural approach to health and maintaining a natural balance within the human body are very important in experiencing energy, vitality, and vibrant health throughout life.

The author recognizes that opinions within scientific and medical fields differ greatly. The purpose of this book is to share educational information and scientific research gathered by the author, scientists, and informed advocates of health and wellbeing using natural methods and resources.

None of the information contained in this book is intended to diagnose, prevent, treat, or cure any disease, nor is it intended to prescribe any of the techniques, materials or concepts presented as a form of treatment for any illness or medical condition. Before beginning any practice of the procedures described in the book, it is highly recommended that you first obtain the consent and advice of licensed health care professional.

The information given in this book should be used for educational purposes only, and not as advice or prescription for specific medical conditions. Responsibility for any action taken as a result of reading this book will lie solely with you. The author assumes no responsibility for the choices you make after you review the information contained herein and your consultation with a licensed healthcare professional.

If you are on medication, do not start taking or using minerals without consulting with your GP since minerals can interfere with medicines.

Module 1 - Course Overview: Resources, Certification, Materials and Equipment, Disclaimer and Therapist Qualification Requirements.

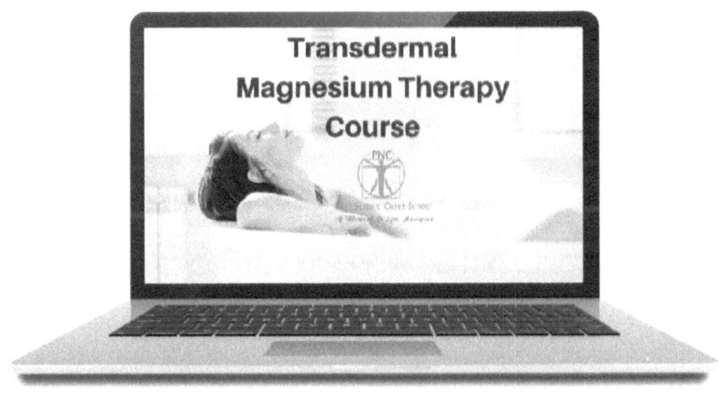

Unit 1 - Course Overview: Resources, Certification and Other Details

Course Overview

Transdermal Magnesium Therapy Course is one of a range of courses developed by Pure Nature Cures School of Mineral & Spa Therapies. The course explores multiple health benefits of magnesium and various transdermal applications of magnesium salts.

Who Is This Course Suitable For?

1. Therapists with a valid Level 3 Anatomy & Physiology + Massage qualifications - to obtain professional insurance and be able to practice professionally.
2. Members of the public who would like to learn the course for their own needs.

Resources

1. Course units
2. Recommended literature & websites.

Certification

The course has been approved by the International Institute of Holistic Therapists. Certification is issued by the Pure Nature Cures School of Mineral & Spa Therapies.

To get certified, you will need to go through our online course and complete the test questions after corresponding units.

Everyone who has completed the course units and quizzes will be issued with a certificate of completion.

If you decide to qualify as a therapist, you will need to complete an add-on unit for therapists, case studies, the practical module and assignments. This will qualify you for the practitioner certificate which you can use to apply for professional insurance.

You will need to make enquiries with your local insurance providers to obtain professional insurance.

Materials & Equipment Needed for the Treatment

1. Magnesium oil, magnesium salts (essential)
2. Other optional components which will be described later in the course.

Unit 2 – Disclaimer

Medical Disclaimer

Neither I personally nor my business makes any representations or guarantees in terms of medical information and research materials described in this Course, express or implied. All information in this Course is presented solely for educational purposes, and not to diagnose or treat any person for any medical symptom, illness or condition.

None of the information, treatments and techniques presented in this Course, in written or oral communication, within our Practical modules, webinars and consultations aims to replace or teach to replace medical diagnosis or treatment. Students are always encouraged to seek medical diagnosis and treatment for any medical problems.

While we aim to present what we believe to be complete, accurate and true information, considering a diversity of views in the medical research field, we cannot guarantee that the information in this Course is always complete, accurate and true. This does exempt us from any liabilities and responsibilities which may not be excluded by applicable legislation.

It is a responsibility of the Reader/ Student/ Therapist to assess their own or their client's health and to make an appropriate decision regarding the suitability of advice or treatment in each particular case. Written consent of the

3rd party must always be obtained before any advice or treatment is provided.

We list some contra-indications to the treatments described in our course materials. However, the list is not exhaustive. The Reader/ Student/ Therapist must always make their assessment of any conditions the 3rd party presents them with and decide whether a treatment is appropriate for themselves or their client.

We will not be held responsible for 3rd party decisions, consultations, treatments or results of these which happen outside the premises and an assigned schedule of the Practical Module Course.

Professional Advice Disclaimer

Neither the information contained within this Course nor communication between the Course Provider/ Book Author/ Business on one hand and Reader/ Student/ Therapist on the other hand, in any form or on any subject

– such as medicine, pharmacology, psychology, finances, commerce, marketing, taxes, accounting, must be regarded nor used as a substitution for professional advice.

Earnings Disclaimer

Neither the information on this Website nor digital or other forms of communication between the Reader/ Student/ Therapist aims to offer any guarantees in terms of potential earnings.

You accept that financial and another type of success depend on a variety of factors, such as knowledge, skills, abilities, dedication, experience, strategies, marketing efforts, networking, the spending power of your potential clients, etc.

As a professional therapist, you are the only person responsible for your earnings and financial success. While we outline revenue potential as a result of the skills you have learned with us, we cannot give any promises or guarantees in this respect, and no statements on this website aim to mislead you in this respect.

Persons under 16

Persons under 16 years of age require their parent's permission to use materials, treatments and techniques, as well as to receive a consultation or a treatment described in this Course. It is the responsibility of a Reader/ Student/ Therapist to ensure that such permission has been obtained before a consultation or a treatment has been provided to a person who is under 16 years of age.

Personal & Professional Responsibility

You agree that you are solely responsible for your own professional (public, product and any other relevant type) liability as a result of your actions. You are the only person responsible for your compliance with the law and regulations in any area of your business.

You agree that by using this Course information and Services, you take full responsibility for your own decisions, actions and results of your actions towards yourself or 3rd parties. You agree to comply with laws and legislation of the country you live in. You are solely responsible for your Professional Indemnity Insurance, National Insurance and taxes.

We highly recommend that you make enquiries about membership of professional organisations and professional liability insurance before you start treating clients. You should always work in the interests of your clients (paying or non-paying) and within the framework of legal and ethical considerations.

All the courses and treatments presented by Pure Nature Cures School of Mineral & Spa Therapies are being marketed as complementary health and beauty courses and treatments, and are not meant to promote or endorse any medical information, or provide diagnosis and/or medical treatment.

Contraindications to Treatments

If you have any medical condition, please address it with a medical professional. The treatments have certain contra-indications, so are not suitable for everyone. See the list of common contra-indications here -
https://courses.purenaturecures.com/contraindications-cautions/

There may be other conditions not listed here which may make a person unsuitable for treatment. If you are unsure, please refer your client to a medical professional. Never conduct treatment without prior consultation to establish a client's suitability for the procedure.

Pure Nature Cures School of Mineral & Spa Therapies offers no diagnosis or treatment of problems of a medical nature, and no guarantees in terms of health benefits described within the Course.

While there are multiple possible benefits to the treatments, they should be seen as part of the integrative approach to health issues rather than a sole option. Any positive results will depend on a combination of factors taken by you or your client, and we cannot and do not offer any guarantees in terms of benefits mentioned within our offers or the course syllabus.

Please let us know if you have any questions, and we will be happy to reply. You can contact us by email: **support@purenaturecures.com**.

For more detailed information about the terms and conditions of using our website and training please see our terms - http://courses.purenaturecures.com/terms/

Unit 3 - Therapist Qualification Requirements

The courses run by the Pure Nature Cures School of Mineral & Spa Therapies are aimed both at therapists and members of the public.

1. Members of the public take our courses to learn about the health benefits of salts, clays and minerals and do treatments on themselves, based on their assessment of their health. In the case of existing health issues, members of the public should always seek medical advice before having a treatment. Even though the majority of people will benefit from the treatments, some people may find them unsuitable. Read about some of the contra-indications and cautions here – https://courses.purenaturecures.com/contraindications-cautions/.

2. Our courses can also be taken by qualified therapists who would like to add new skills to their portfolio. To be considered qualified, a therapist needs to have a Level 3 Anatomy & Physiology and Body Massage Diploma.

3. While all the students will be issued with the Certificate of Completion, only qualified therapists will receive a Practitioner Certificate which will allow them to apply for Practitioner insurance and treat members of the public.

4. We cannot guarantee that the qualification we offer will be accepted by insurers in the country of your residence, due to variations regarding requirements for complementary therapies. Please make enquiries with your local insurance providers.

5. To qualify as a therapist, you will need to sign up for the add-on short course for therapists which covers subjects such as hygiene, professional issues, as well as case studies.

6. The optional practical one-day module is offered to therapists in the UK & Northern Ireland, as well as to those who can travel to the UK for the course.

Module 2 - Magnesium - The Mineral of Life

Unit 1 - The Importance of Magnesium for Health

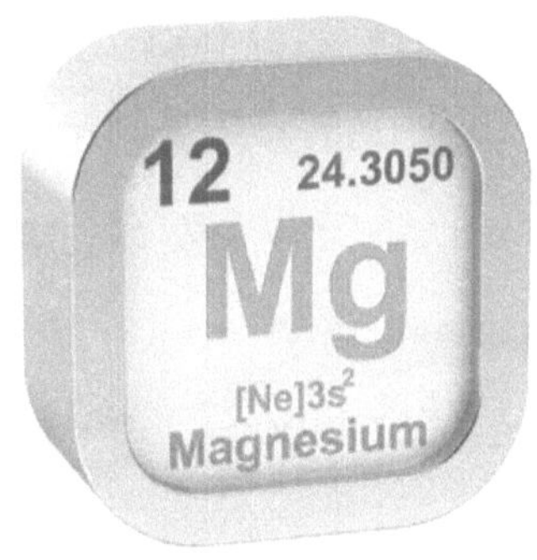

Magnesium is rightly called a "miracle mineral". There are few minerals which attract so much attention and instigate so much scientific research. The reason is that it not only participates in over 300 biochemical reactions in the body but helps maintain so many bodily functions, such as the normal muscle and nerve function, steady heart rhythm, normal blood pressure, healthy immune system and strong bones. It also helps to maintain blood sugar at normal levels. It plays a vital role in preventing heart disease, diabetes, cancer, osteoporosis and a whole range of other problems.

Magnesium is the **fourth most abundant element in the body**. About half of the total body magnesium is found in bones. The other half is found mostly inside cells of body tissues and organs. Only 1% of magnesium is found in the blood where it plays a vital role, so the body works very hard to keep the blood magnesium levels constant.

"...An important participant in enzyme processes which ensure protein biosynthesis and carbohydrate metabolism. It is also very important for the nervous and muscular systems, helps to maintain the healthy tone of the blood vessels. Magnesium is a 'calming' element for the nervous system slowing down the brain activity. It expands the blood vessels and is a natural diuretic. Generally, it is vital for all body systems and processes.

The adult requirement for magnesium is 350-500mg per day. Fresh green vegetables, seafood, soybeans, special nutritional yeasts, seeds, apples and whole grains are rich sources." Read more about the role of magnesium in the body -

http://www.traceminerals.com/research/magnesium.html

Magnesium has been found to:

- Stimulate protein/fat metabolism
- Reduce inflammation by lowering the levels of histamine and serotonin (mediators of inflammation)
- Speed up rehabilitation processes in the body
- Increase testosterone levels and sperm production
- Strengthen immunity
- Slow down ageing

- Reduce cholesterol levels in the blood
- Improve the functioning of the musculoskeletal system
- Reduce blood pressure
- Significantly reduce heart disease and mortality
- Lower the incidence of cancer
- Improve the functioning of the Nervous System
- Reduce the effects of stress
- Increase phagocytosis
- Speed up tissue regeneration
- Improve skin condition
- Speed up body metabolism
- Raise energy levels (magnesium is the essential mineral in the production of energy)
- Promote weight loss.

It has been proved to be a:

- Sedative

- Anti-inflammatory

- Bactericidal / fungicidal

- Circulation booster

- Analgesic

- Immune regulator.

Further Reading

1. Magnesium -
http://www.traceminerals.com/research/magnesium.htm

2. Magnesium -
http://ods.od.nih.gov/factsheets/magnesium.asp

3. Magnesium -
http://umm.edu/health/medical/altmed/supplement/magnesium.

Unit 2 - Causes & Signs of Magnesium Deficiency

What Happens When We Become Magnesium-Deficient?

Magnesium deficiency is more common than we realise. According to American nutritionists, an average adult needs 200mg more magnesium per day than what is obtained from a diet. The fact is, that dietary magnesium is not sufficient in providing the body with this important mineral. Magnesium deficiency can be explained by many factors, with the main reasons being depletion of soil in minerals.

"Early signs of magnesium deficiency include loss of appetite, nausea, vomiting, fatigue, and weakness. As magnesium deficiency worsens, numbness, tingling, muscle contractions and cramps, seizures, personality changes, abnormal heart rhythms, and coronary spasms can occur."

http://ods.od.nih.gov/factsheets/magnesium.asp

Magnesium deficiency may also lead to:

- Loss of energy

- Slowing down of metabolism

- Disturbances in calcium and potassium balance in the blood

- High cholesterol level

- A formation of cholesterol plaque

- Kidney and gallbladder stones

- Arthritis

- Anxiety

- Depression

- Muscle tension

- Joint pain

- Acidosis

- Nervous tension

- Insomnia

- Diabetes

- Osteoporosis

- Chronic fatigue

- Poor immunity

- Menstrual pain

- Fertility problems.

What causes magnesium deficiency?

Magnesium deficiency is commonly caused by and associated with the following factors:

- Stress - physical and mental
- Certain medications (e.g. insulin, diuretics, some asthma medications, birth control pills, corticosteroids, blood pressure control medicines, etc)
- Extreme physical training
- Chemical toxins getting into the body from the environment
- Excessive intake of sodium chloride (table salt), sugar, caffeine, alcohol, nicotine, cocaine, fizzy drinks (especially colas)
- Prolonged intense sweating, due to exercise or illness

- Diarrhoea
- Malnutrition. This involves not only insufficient food intake but also the consumption of nutrient-poor foods
- Consuming food products which come from magnesium-deficient soils
- Drinking water which is high in potassium
- Prolonged physical exercise
- Diabetes
- Obesity
- Kidney disease
- Malabsorption
- Digestive disorders
- Crohn's disease
- Chemotherapy and radiotherapy
- Liver disease
- Inflammation
- Serious injuries
- Excessive intake of vitamin D
- Excessive consumption of dairy products (especially cheese)
- Pancreatitis

- Severe burns.

Further Reading

1. Magnesium Deficiency Symptoms & Diagnosis, Mark Sircus.
http://drsircus.com/medicine/magnesium/magnesium-deficiency-symptoms-diagnosis
2. What Causes Magnesium Deficiency?
http://www.magnesiumoil.org.uk/what-causes-magnesium-deficiency/

Unit 3 - Dangers of Magnesium Deficiency to Health

Here are some conditions which may develop as a result of the long-term magnesium deficiency:

- **Anxiety and panic attacks.** Magnesium helps to keep hormones in balance, and adrenal stress under control.

- Serotonin, the hormone responsible for mood regulation, is dependent on magnesium levels being at the optimal level in the body at all times.
- **Impaired detoxification.** Removal of toxic elements such as lead and aluminium from the body requires the presence of sufficient levels of magnesium.
- Magnesium is needed for insulin secretion, to help metabolise sugar. Without magnesium insulin cannot transfer glucose into cells, which leads to the build-up of both glucose and insulin in the blood, leading to tissue damage.
- **Metabolic syndrome.** This condition is partly due to insufficient magnesium levels in the body, which leads to insulin not being activated, glucose not delivered to the body cells, and energy not being produced. This slows down the body metabolism. It is closely connected with diabetes.
- This is also partly a result of magnesium deficiency, due to malnutrition and slow metabolism. To add to this, there is a permanent cycle of anxiety-triggered overeating, which is both caused by and leads to

magnesium deficiency. Of course, one cannot just blame the low magnesium level for obesity, but it plays a big role in developing the condition.

- Magnesium deficiency causes slowing down of bowel movement and constipation, which leads to an increase in toxicity and nutrient deficiency.

- **Muscle cramps.** Magnesium is the ultimate natural relaxant. Without sufficient magnesium in the blood, calcium takes over leading to calcification of tissues and cramps.

- **Musculoskeletal problems.** Aches, pains, muscle tension are all made worse where there is not enough magnesium is present in the body. This happens due to insufficient relaxation of the muscles due to a magnesium-calcium imbalance, which can lead to chronic tension, joint problems, inflammation and other musculoskeletal conditions, such as back problems, osteoarthritis, frozen shoulder, RSA, and more.

- Blood contains both calcium and magnesium, and a healthy ratio (approximately 1:1) is important to ensure bone health. Contrary to popular belief, just taking calcium and vitamin D, without supplementing magnesium, may worsen the condition, and lead to other problems.

- **Tooth decay.** Insufficient magnesium causes an imbalance of phosphorus and calcium in the saliva which leads to tooth decay.

- **Blood clots.** Magnesium plays an important role in keeping the blood thin. Magnesium deficiency leads to thickening of the blood, and the formation of blood clots, which is a potentially fatal condition.

- **Arterial plaque/ atherosclerosis.** Magnesium is necessary to keep the optimal calcium-magnesium ratio in the blood. When there is not enough magnesium, this ratio gets compromised, leading to the formation of arterial plaque, which consists of excessive blood calcium, proteins and fat. This is also a potentially fatal condition.

- **PMS/ PMT - premenstrual syndrome/ tension** are often directly linked to magnesium deficiency.

- **Pre-eclampsia, eclampsia and premature contractions -** all of these dangerous conditions are directly caused by a magnesium-calcium imbalance (too much calcium, very low magnesium).

- Magnesium is the "energy" mineral. It is the spark needed to convert glucose into energy. Magnesium is also used in the production of enzymes. When there is not enough magnesium in the body, energy does not get produced leading to fatigue, sometimes chronic.

- **Hypertension (high blood pressure)**. Being a natural relaxant, magnesium is needed to keep the blood vessels supple and open. It also regulates the amount of calcium and cholesterol in the blood. If the magnesium level is low, the blood starts circulating too much calcium and cholesterol - ideal materials for plaque formation. Plus, insufficient magnesium leading too much calcium leads to inflammations and rigidity of the tissues, including blood vessels. Inflammation can lead to damage to the blood vessels, which can result in the formation of scar tissue. The plaque has more chances of forming in the area of scar tissue. Once the plaque is formed, it keeps growing, and eventually, the opening narrows down, so blood pressure goes up. It's like with a garden hose - try pinching or bending it to restrict the water flow and see what happens.

- **Heart disease.** Magnesium deficiency is often associated with heart disease. Doctors have been using magnesium injections for cardiac arrest and arrhythmia for a long time. The heart muscle, like any other muscles in the body, depends on a continuous blood supply which delivers nutrients and oxygen. Where there is not enough magnesium, a build-up of arterial plaque may lead to the constriction of the blood vessels supplying the heart muscle, and even blockage which can result in a heart attack. A magnesium sulphate injection is the first aid remedy in such cases, and doctors working in accident and emergency departments know it all too well.

- **Hypoglycaemia** - low blood sugar level. Blood sugar levels depend on sufficient levels of magnesium in the body which is needed for the regulation of insulin activity. Insufficient magnesium can lead not only to a build-up of glucose but to hypoglycaemia as well.

- Insufficient magnesium in the body increases bronchial spasm, as well as histamine production.
- There is a direct link between magnesium deficiency and an allergic reaction since magnesium manages histamine production and response within the body.
- **Kidney disease.** Magnesium deficiency can lead to abnormal lipid levels and blood sugar control, and this can lead to kidney failure.
- **Headache & migraine.** Low magnesium levels lead to narrowing of blood vessels and muscle spasms, which can lead to restriction of blood flow to the brain. The other factor contributing to headaches and migraines is that serotonin does not get produced in sufficient amounts.
- **Nerve disorders.** Nerve tissue depends on magnesium for its health. Magnesium is needed to transmit nerve signals between the brain and other organs and tissues since it activates calcium. Insufficient magnesium leads to peripheral nerve problems, as well as dysfunctions of the central nervous system.

These are only some conditions caused by magnesium deficiency. All of them require an increased and consistent magnesium supplementation, and oral supplementation is normally not enough.

Dr Calolyn Dean lists the following conditions which develop in cases of magnesium deficiency or and require magnesium supplementation:

"Acid reflux, Adrenal fatigue, Alzheimer's disease, Angina, Anxiety and panic attacks, Arthritis, Asthma, Atherosclerosis, Blood clots, Bowel disease, Brain dysfunction, Bruxism or teeth grinding, Cholesterol elevation, cystitis, Depression, Detoxification, Diabetes, Fatigue, Headaches, Heart disease, Hypertension, Hypoglycemia, Indigestion, Inflammation, Insomnia, IBS, Kidney disease, Kidney stones, Migraine, Muscoluskeletal conditions: (muscle cramps, fibrositis, fibromyalgia, GI spasms, tension headaches, muscle spams or muscle contractions in any muscle of the body, chronic neck and back pain, jaw tension), Nerve problems – Neuralgia, Neuritis, Neuropathy (burning pain, muscle weakness, numbness paralysis, pins and needles, seizures and convulsions, tingling twitching, vertigo, confusion),

Obstetrical and gynaecological problems (PMS, dysmenorrhea, female infertility, premature contractions, pre-eclampsia and eclampsia, cerebral palsy, sudden infant death syndrome, male infertility), Osteoporosis, Parkinson's disease, Raynaud's syndrome, Sports injuries, Sports recovery, Tempromandibular joint syndrome, Tongue biting, Tooth decay." http://drcarolyndean.com/

Further Reading

"The Magnesium Miracle", by Dr Carolyn Dean.

Module 3 - Magnesium for Pain Management

Unit 1 - Anatomy of a Nerve Cell. Types and Causes of Pain.

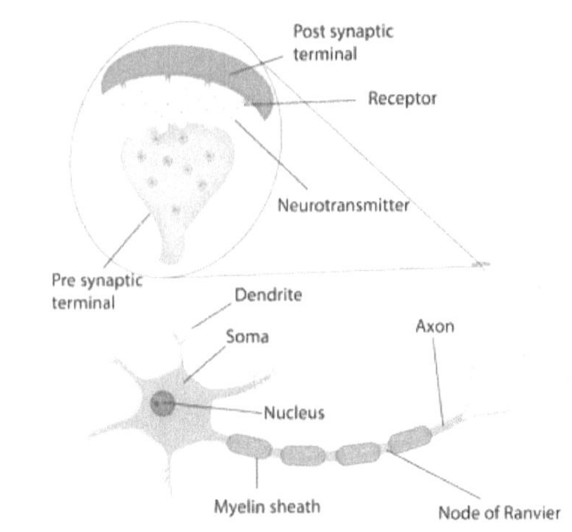

Anatomy of a Nerve Cell

Pain is a signal that something is not right. Its main goal is to protect the body from harm. The nervous system can normally tell the difference between the pain signals which may be harmful and those which are not, instinctively, by-passing the cognitive part of the brain.

The nervous system consists of two major parts:

1. The central nervous system which includes the brain and the spinal cord
2. The peripheral nervous system comprising all the other nerves.

The main building block of the nervous system is a **nerve cell or neuron**. It consists of:

1. Cell body (Soma) - the main part of a neuron where the nucleus is found.
2. Dendrites - projections radiating from the neuron in all directions. A single neuron can have up to 200 of them. They receive signals to the nerve.

3. Axon, which is sometimes covered with myelin sheath - the fatty coating which protects the axon and speeds up nerve signal transmission.

4. Synaptic end bulb - the swelling at the end of the nerve cell which contains the neurotransmitter.

5. Synapse - a space which separates the end bulb from an adjacent nerve cell or dendrite.

6. The node of Ranvier - a gap in the myelin sheath which helps the conduction of the nerve impulse.

"Nerve impulses travel along neurons in the form of electrical signals. These signals cross the synapses (tiny gaps) between one neuron and the next in the chemical form before being transmitted again in electrical form. Signals are also chemically transmitted to other target cells, such as those in muscles, which make appropriate responses."

http://www.aviva.co.uk/health-insurance/home-of-health/medical-centre/medical-encyclopedia/entry/structure-and-function-nerve-cells/

Pain and response to it are transmitted to and from the brain via nerve cells. Types of nerves include sensory and motor nerves. Sensory nerves carry messages from the body to the brain. The response is carried from the brain to the body by the motor nerves. It is the sensory nerves that trigger the reflex that pulls us away from pain.

Most sensory and motor nerves are enclosed in a myelin sheath that acts as a conductor for impulses in the nerve fibre. The signals between neurons are electric by nature and are transmitted from one cell to other thanks to neurotransmitters, and there is a range of these in the body.

Types & Causes of Pain

Somatic Pain is sharp and localised. It is felt in the skin, muscles, joints and ligaments. The nerve receptors with this type of pain are sensitive to pressure, temperature, stretch, vibration. They are also sensitive to inflammation, as would happen if you cut yourself, sprain something that causes tissue damage. It also includes pain as a result of lack of oxygen, as in ischemic muscle cramps.

Visceral Pain is felt in the internal organs and main body cavities - the thorax (lungs and heart), abdomen (bowel, spleen, liver and kidneys), and the pelvis (ovaries, bladder, and the womb). The pain receptors sense inflammation, stretch and ischemia (oxygen starvation). Visceral pain is harder to localise, and the sensation is more like a deep dull ache. This is why pain is often referred to as "ache". It can also radiate to other body organs.

Nerve Pain (Neuropathic Pain) comes from within the nervous system itself. You may have heard people referring to a pinched or trapped nerve. The pain can originate from the nerves between the tissues and the spinal cord (peripheral nervous system) and the nerves between the spinal cord and the brain (central nervous system). It can be caused by nerve degeneration, for example as a result of a stroke or oxygen starvation. It may also be due to a trapped nerve, which puts pressure on it. Nerve infection in the case of shingles, or a torn/slipped intervertebral disc can cause this kind of pain.

Sympathetic Pain The sympathetic nervous system controls the blood flow to our skin and muscles, perspiration, and the speed of functioning of the peripheral nervous system. Sympathetic pain happens after a fracture or a soft tissue injury of the limbs. There are no specific pain receptors with this type of pain.

As with neuropathic pain, the nerve is injured, becomes unstable and fires off random, abnormal signals to the brain, which interprets them as pain. With this type of pain, the skin and the area around the injury become extremely sensitive. The pain can virtually immobilise a limb, which if lasting too long can cause other problems, such as muscle wasting, osteoporosis, arthritis, and joint stiffness.

Unit 2 - Magnesium for Muscle Cramps

Cramps of any kind are sudden, involuntary contractions of muscles or muscles. Most common cramps are experienced in the calf muscles and the soles of the feet and occur during the night or while at rest.

Cramps can also affect other muscles in the body in people of any age group. Stomach cramps are quite common, especially with women of reproductive age.

There may be various causes for cramps to happen. Scientific research has not identified a precise reason for muscle cramps. However, it may be due to the nerves controlling the muscles rather than the muscles themselves.

Leg cramps can be caused by over-exertion of the muscles, structural disorders (such as flat feet), prolonged sitting, standing on a hard surface, or dehydration. Less common causes include diabetes, hypoglycemia, anaemia, thyroid and endocrine dysfunction, Parkinson's and certain medications.

Low levels of certain minerals acting as electrolytes in the body - they include magnesium, potassium, sodium and calcium - have long been linked to leg cramps. It especially affects long-distance runners and cyclists. Diuretics can also cause leg cramps. Pregnant women are also more susceptible to leg cramps.

"Canadian doctors have found that magnesium supplements can alleviate muscle cramps. In severe cases, magnesium has been provided intravenously and this has led to the relief of symptoms within 24 hours. Many cases of muscle cramps are caused by low concentrations of magnesium in the blood... The reason why it helps is due to diuretic medications or strenuous exercise. When taken orally, it seems that magnesium glucoheptonate or magnesium gluconate works best". Bilbey, Douglas L, Prabhakaran V.M. Muscle cramps and magnesium deficiency: case reports. Canadian Family Physician. July

Transdermal Magnesium Therapy Course for Clinic & Home Use

http://www.internethealthlibrary.com/Health-problems/Muscle%20cramps%20-%20researchDiet&Lifestyle.htm

Dr John Briffa says: "I remember once attending a nutritional therapy course for doctors in the US, in which one of the facilitators (Dr Jonathan Wright) said, "If it spasms, think magnesium" (or something similar). And this sage piece of advice was based on the idea that low levels of magnesium in the body tend to cause a muscle to go into spasm. This might include so-called 'smooth' muscle in, say, the digestive tract, bladder on in the walls of the arteries. It might also include 'skeletal' muscle, say, in the legs. Ever since hearing learning this, I've used magnesium generally very effectively to treat conditions like muscular cramps, 'restless legs', irritable bladder syndrome and oesophageal spasm".

http://www.drbriffa.com/blog/2009/12/29/a-case-of-oesophageal-spasm-and-the-unproven-treatment-that-helped-it/

To prevent cramps from happening, magnesium, potassium and sodium levels have to be monitored - especially in people who lose a lot of fluids due to exercise, excessive sweating, vomiting or diarrhoea. Magnesium is best absorbed by the body when applied on the skin. It is the quickest method too.

Unit 3 – Managing Pain with Magnesium

Magnesium is one of the most powerful natural relaxants in nature. It also has a profound effect on the functioning of the nervous system. Without sufficient magnesium, nerves start firing signals too easily with even a minor stimulus. Noises become too loud, lights too bright, emotions exaggerated. Magnesium is known to regulate or inhibit many nerve receptors. It acts like water on fire cooling down the nervous system.

Magnesium also appears to be able to affect the nervous system by regulating the release of hormones, which occurs due to many different forms of stress. "Without enough magnesium, serotonin flows unchecked,

constricting blood vessels and releasing other pain-producing chemicals such as substance P and prostaglandins, he says. Normal magnesium levels not only prevent the release of these pain-producing substances but also stop their effects, says Dr Altura."
http://www.mgwater.com/prev1801.shtml

Unfortunately, it is very difficult to determine magnesium deficiency using a blood test, since blood serum level does not reflect the amount of magnesium in the tissues. This is the reason it often gets overlooked, and unnoticed, with dire consequences to health. Also, it is difficult to achieve optimal magnesium levels via oral supplementation.

The reason for it is that magnesium is not easily absorbed by the digestive system. If digestion is compromised due to an IBS, gluten intolerance, or leaky gut, then supplementation becomes an even greater challenge.

Further Reading

1. Inflammation & Pain Management with Magnesium. http://drsircus.com/medicine/magnesium/inflammation-and-systemic-stress
2. Magnesium Treats Fibromyalgia Pain. http://www.fmnetnews.com/latest-news/magnesium-treats-fibromyalgia-pain

Module 4 - Magnesium for Stress & Stress-Related Problems

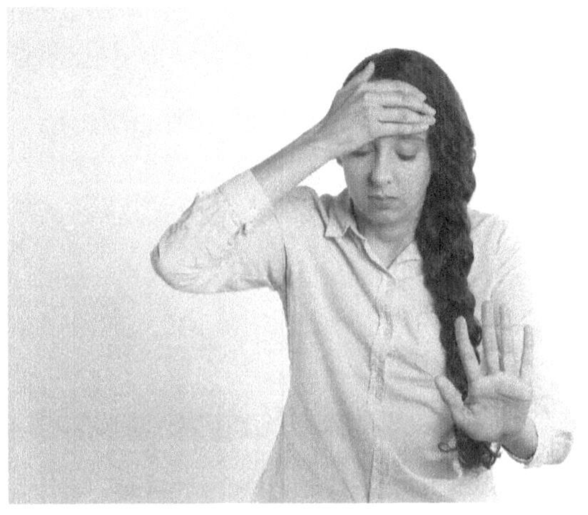

Unit 1 - Definition of Stress. Acute Stress - Symptoms & Consequences. Repeated Acute Stress.

In simple terms, **stress is the body-mind response to real or perceived events and situations in its surroundings**. It can be caused both by what is perceived as "good" or "bad". The "good" factors include what we find exciting, stimulating, highly pleasurable.

For example, a jump from a plane with a parachute - it is a stressful activity, but in most cases exciting at the same time. The "bad" stressors are the ones which cause distress to the mind and body - for example, an attack from somebody, real or perceived.

Acute Stress

This is a short-lived type of stress. The body responds to it with a **"fight or flight" strategy**. This kind of response causes fast changes in the body, to ensure its survival. A release of adrenaline and other related hormones mobilises the body resources within a short time.

The limb muscles contract, the heart starts pumping the blood a lot faster, blood flow to the limbs and major organs increases, to make sure that the body can either fight or flee. This is a biological response which in dangerous situations saves lives. However, in many cases danger is perceived, rather than present, and a lot of people get acutely stressed over things which are non-life-threatening (e.g. road rage).

Acute stress is accountable for most cases of cardiac arrest (heart attack) and **can be very dangerous if there are long-term chronic problems present in the body**. The other type of acute stress involves **pleasant activities and events** - a birth of a child, moving home, doing something for fun and excitement (e.g. a ski jump). This stress is short-lived, but can still disrupt the body processes.

Common symptoms and consequences

- A sudden rise in blood pressure
- Muscle tension, cramps
- Disruption of the digestive processes
- Increased risk of cardiac arrest
- Increased risk of stroke
- Disruption of the endocrine system
- Flaring up of chronic conditions

- Long-term physical and psychological problems.

Repeated acute stress

This kind of stress involves **repetition of stressful situations and events**. It also describes the mind's perception of the environment as threatening and hostile, with the corresponding reaction. Like with acute stress, it can be real (e.g. a soldier or a civilian in a war zone), or perceived (a teenager seeing the world as a deeply hostile environment, with no way out). This is a **more dangerous kind of stress** since the body and mind balance get repeatedly disrupted, with hormones wreaking havoc with the body systems.

Common symptoms and consequences

- Anxiety
- Depression
- Wearing down of all the body systems
- A build-up of toxins in the body

- Stroke
- Cardiac problems
- Blood pressure problems
- Cancer

Although acute stress is less likely to cause long-term damage as chronic stress does, it is more devastating for people whose health is already under par - especially for people with circulation/blood pressure problems and heart disease.

Acute stress can lead to a sudden spike in blood pressure which can, in turn, result in a heart attack or a stroke. So training oneself to respond to such situations calmly and constructively can save a life.

Unit 2 - Chronic Stress - Symptoms & Consequences

Chronic Stress

This is the silent killer which destroys the body and mind consistently, over some time. The most possible causes are one's response to financial hardship, relationship problems, a feeling of being stuck in the rut due to entrenched beliefs and inflexible mindset, long-term illness, lack of help, loneliness, bullying, uninspiring home and work environment.

The damage which long-term stress causes to the body is often devastating. People who are continually exposed to chronic stress are much more likely to suffer from poor health, which can lead to health problems, heart disease, cancer and premature death.

Common symptoms and consequences of chronic stress

- High cholesterol level in the blood, leading to clogged up and rigid arteries (atherosclerosis and arteriosclerosis)
- Over-eating, leading to obesity

- Obesity caused by an accumulation of toxins in the body
- Type 2 diabetes due to insulin resistance from the cells
- Inflammation of the joints (arthritis, rheumatism)
- Blood pressure abnormalities
- Chronic anxiety
- Depression
- Passive aggression
- Sudden seemingly unexplained episodes of a panic attack and acute anxiety
- Chronic Fatigue Syndrome
- Fibromyalgia
- Kidney disease
- Psoriasis, dermatitis, eczema
- Acne and other skin problems
- Allergies
- Stroke
- Poor immunity
- Disturbed sleep
- Headaches, migraine
- Depression

- Alcoholism
- Drug abuse
- Other addictions
- Cancer.

Long-term cholesterol production which happens when a person goes through prolonged periods of stress causes inflammations and undermines immunity to disease. It also uses up the body magnesium resources, since so much of this mineral is required to produce hormones responding to stress, as well as just to keep the body alive and brain functioning. This is why magnesium supplementation during such periods is so important. Not only does it help the body to cope with stress, but it also helps prevent a serious illness from setting in.

Unit 3 – Stress - the Magnesium Link

Topping up magnesium levels through the skin is one of the quickest and most effective ways to deal with stress. Let's remember that magnesium takes part in over 350 body processes. It is needed for the production of hormones and enzymes which deal with stress and its effects.

No wonder that when we experience acute stress or go through prolonged periods of chronic stress, the demand for it becomes very high. Magnesium is used up and gets depleted fast if we don't top it up, which puts the body under even more stress, preventing it from performing vital functions.

Because most food is low in magnesium, and many of us rely on convenience food, the body simply gets starved of this vital mineral. We start experiencing pain in the chest, cannot sleep well, become anxious, and eventually depressed. Our body muscles become tense. Cramps become a regular occurrence. The stomach becomes too acidic, which may lead to irritable bowel, gastritis and even ulcers.

Apart from using up most of the magnesium reserves, with chronic stress, the body starts producing too much cortisol (a hormone which helps the body adjust to stress), the side-effects of which include chronic inflammation, raised blood sugar level and therefore production and release of insulin, which increases the risk of diabetes.

A study has found researching a link between stress, magnesium deficiency and the immune response has found out that "Mg deficiency results in a stress effect and increased susceptibility to physiological damage produced by stress. Stress activates the sympathetic nervous system and renin-angiotensin-aldosterone axis resulting in increased oxidative stress.

Aldosteronism is immunostimulatory, as is commonly seen in congestive heart failure. The inflammatory syndrome induces mechanisms dependent on cytosolic calcium activation. These interrelationships support that the Mg effect on intracellular calcium homeostasis may be a common link between stress and inflammation".
http://www.omicsonline.org/magnesium-influence-on-stress-and-immune-function-in-exercise-2161-0673.1000111.pdf

High cholesterol level and formation of arterial plaques are almost inevitable in cases of prolonged stress. Comfort eating contributes to weight gain, which in turn increases the risk of diabetes, heart disease and cancer. So it becomes a vicious circle which with time gets harder and harder to break.

It is amazing how simply by including magnesium in the diet things begin to turn for the better. Of course, magnesium alone won't do it. We need to take a whole range of steps to break this cycle and regain our health. Exercise, good nutrition, plenty of water, learning to deal with stressful situations and creating a stress-free environment at home and at work all need to be considered. But topping up magnesium levels in the body will bring almost immediate relief (depending on the method of supplementation).

Doctors have known and used magnesium (and still do) to pull a person from an emergency, such as an irregular heartbeat and heart attack by injecting magnesium intravenously. This is a lifesaver for dying patients. So why not use this relatively cheap and very effective mineral to help ourselves which would help us avoid emergencies?

Transdermal magnesium salt application is the quickest way to top up magnesium level quickly, literally within minutes, bringing instant relaxation. Taken orally, magnesium is also a great help, but it takes time to start working, and some magnesium may get through the body unabsorbed. So every person should keep magnesium oil or magnesium salt at home at all times, and of course, remember to use it regularly.

Module 5 - Stress, Obesity & Diabetes – How They Are Linked to Each Other and Magnesium

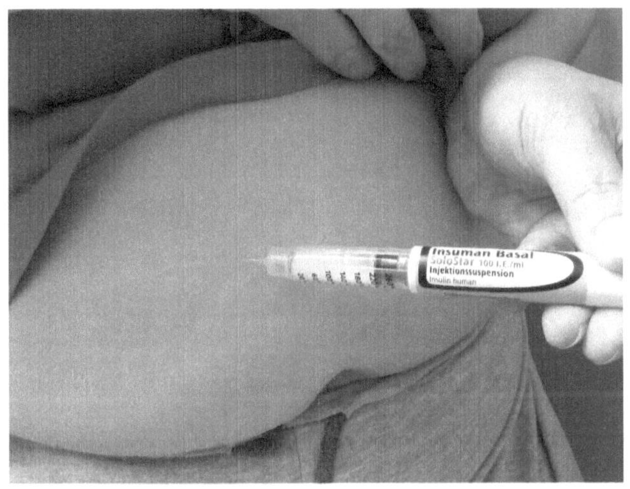

Unit 1 - Magnesium Deficiency, Obesity & Diabetes - How Are They Connected?

With the obesity levels reaching record levels in the UK and other parts of the world, it is essential to mention how important a role magnesium plays in weight management.

Magnesium plays a crucial part in the production and storage of energy, by activating ATP (adenosine triphosphate) – the molecule which stores energy in the body. This is what Dr Carolyn Dean, an authority on the subject of magnesium for health, says:

"Magnesium and B-complex vitamins are excellent examples of energy nutrients because they activate enzymes that control digestion, absorption, and the utilisation of proteins, fats, and carbohydrates. Enzymes cannot be produced and nutrients cannot be utilised, which means that energy cannot be manufactured and stored in the body without magnesium.

Magnesium deficiency is closely associated with obesity and related conditions. Type 2 diabetes is one such condition which is on the rise both in the developed and developing the world. It has been established that type 2 diabetes responds very well to magnesium supplementation. Magnesium is needed for production and utilisation of insulin by the cells. "Low magnesium, widely recognised as a marker for diabetes, occurs in up to 40% of diabetic patients.

Lack of magnesium increases the risk of cardiovascular disease, eye symptoms, and nerve damage in diabetics, whereas supplementation can prevent them. Most importantly for diabetics, magnesium is a necessary cofactor in the production of energy from sugar stores in the muscles and liver." (The Miracle of Magnesium, Carolyn Dean, M.D., N.D.).

Magnesium deficiency also creates cellular resistance to insulin, since insulin opens the cells to glucose only in the presence of sufficient magnesium, so the cell does not receive glucose, and cannot produce energy. The glucose, in this case, accumulates in the blood causing irrevocable damage to the body organs, blood vessels, nerves and other systems.

Since obesity is often interlinked with diabetes and pre-diabetic conditions, it is very important to ensure sufficient magnesium intake to address obesity and for management and prevention of diabetes. Of course, magnesium alone will not solve the problem of obesity. A lot of factors, such as correct nutrition, exercise, psychological problems need to be addressed. However, if magnesium deficiency is not addressed all these measures may produce only a limited and short-lived result.

As well as eating traditionally magnesium-rich foods, magnesium needs to be supplemented both orally and transdermally to produce a visible impact. Spraying or rubbing magnesium chloride solution all over the body daily, taking magnesium baths or even footbaths can replenish magnesium levels quickly, with powerful results which can show almost immediately.

Further Reading

1. Magnesium - the Weight Loss Cure.
http://www.naturalnews.com/036049_magnesium_weight_loss_cure.html

2. Magnesium, Leptin & Obesity, Dr Sircus. http://drsircus.com/medicine/magnesium/magnesium-leptin-obesity

3. Magnesium for Weight Loss. http://www.med-health.net/Magnesium-For-Weight-Loss.html

Unit 2 - The Link Between Stress, Magnesium Deficiency & Obesity

We are used to common thinking that when we get stressed we lose appetite, and therefore weight. Well, yes and no. The relationship between stress and obesity is a lot more complex than this. To understand it, we need to look at the nature of 3 different types of stress, and how they affect the body.

Correlation between Stress and Obesity

Here are conclusions of 2 scientific studies which explain what happens in the body as a result of chronic stress, and how it leads to obesity:

1. "The effects of adrenal corticosteroids on subsequent adrenocorticotropin secretion are complex. Acutely (within hours), **glucocorticoids** (GCs) directly inhibit further activity in the hypothalamo–pituitary–adrenal axis, but the **chronic actions (across days) of these steroids on the brain are directly excitatory.** Chronically high concentrations of GCs act in three ways that are functionally congruent. (*i*) GCs increase the expression of corticotropin-releasing factor (CRF) mRNA in the central nucleus of the amygdala, a critical node in the emotional brain.

CRF enables recruitment of a chronic stress-response network. (*ii*) **GCs increase the salience of pleasurable or compulsive activities (ingesting sucrose, fat, and drugs, or wheel-running).** This motivates ingestion of "comfort food." (*iii*) GCs act systemically to **increase abdominal fat depots.** This allows an increased signal of abdominal energy stores to inhibit catecholamines in the brainstem and CRF expression in hypothalamic neurons regulating adrenocorticotropin.

Chronic stress, together with high GC concentrations, usually decreases body weight gain in rats; by contrast, **in stressed or depressed humans chronic stress induces either increased comfort food intake and body weight gain** or decreased intake and body weight loss. Comfort food ingestion that produces abdominal obesity, decreases CRF mRNA in the hypothalamus of rats.

Depressed people who overeat have decreased cerebrospinal CRF, catecholamine concentrations, and hypothalamo–pituitary–adrenal activity. We propose that **people eat comfort food in an attempt to reduce the activity in the chronic stress-response network with its attendant anxiety.** These mechanisms, determined in rats, may explain some of the epidemics of obesity occurring in our society."
http://www.pnas.org/content/100/20/11696.short

2. "Although stressors generally reduce the intake of boring but healthy foods (chow for rats), **both acute and repeated restraint stress increase the intake of**

highly palatable calories (32% sucrose, lard), when they are available. This behavioural effect is mediated by elevated glucocorticoids and depends on the accompanying increase in circulating insulin concentrations. In the periphery, whereas glucocorticoids mobilize stored calories and greatly increase the rate of gluconeogenesis, insulin counteracts the effects of glucocorticoids, abetting caloric storage. Together, **increasing concentrations of both hormones increase adipose storage**, at the expense of peripheral protein stores when there is not an overall gain in body weight. "
http://www.endocrine-abstracts.org/ea/0019/ea0019s10.htm

3. "In population studies, adrenal hormones show strong statistical associations to centralization of body fat as well as to obesity. There is considerable evidence from clinical to cellular and molecular studies that **elevated cortisol**, particularly when combined with secondary inhibition of sex steroids and growth hormone secretions, is causing accumulation of fat in visceral adipose tissues as well as metabolic abnormalities (The Metabolic Syndrome).

Hypertension is probably due to parallel activation of the central sympathetic nervous system...

3. Glucocorticoid exposure is also followed by increased food intake and 'leptin resistant' obesity, perhaps disrupting the balance between leptin and neuropeptide Y to the advantage of the latter. The consequence might be 'stress-eating', which, however, is a poorly defined entity. Factors activating the stress centres in humans include psychosocial and socioeconomic handicaps, depressive and anxiety traits, alcohol and smoking, with some differences in profile between personalities and genders. Polymorphisms have been defined in several genes associated with the cascade of events along the stress axes."

http://onlinelibrary.wiley.com/

4. "Stress is experienced by animals and humans daily and many individuals experience cycles of stress and recovery throughout the day. If we consume larger and less frequent meals, the conditions are favourable for weight gain-- especially in the abdomen. We know that belly fat, as well as stress, contributes to the development of the

cardiovascular disease, immune dysfunction and other metabolic disorders."
http://www.the-aps.org/mm/hp/Audiences/Public-Press/For-the-Press/releases/10/27.html

Stress, Obesity and Magnesium Deficiency - Studies

Magnesium deficiency is both the consequence and reason for stress and weight gain. When in the state of either acute or chronic stress, magnesium levels get severely depleted, since it takes part in so many processes associated with stress response - production of multiple hormones and neurotransmitters being just some of them. So, the body needs a large amount of magnesium to be able to cope with challenging situations efficiently. If the body resources are depleted already before it is required, then the need becomes even more acute, since the stressful situation depletes it even more. Unless the problem of magnesium deficiency is addressed urgently, the body systems will keep being compromised as a result.

Results of some studies:

1. "...Low magnesium status has been associated with numerous pathological conditions characterized as having a chronic inflammatory stress component. In humans, deficient magnesium intakes are mostly marginal to moderate (approximately 50% to <100% of the recommended dietary allowance)... This suggestion may have significance in obesity, which is characterized as having a chronic low-grade inflammation component and an increased incidence of low magnesium status. "
http://onlinelibrary.wiley.com/

2. A study conducted on obese children with insulin resistance concluded: " The association between magnesium deficiency and IR is present during childhood. Serum magnesium deficiency in obese children may be secondary to decreased dietary magnesium intake. Magnesium supplementation or increased intake of magnesium-rich foods may be an important tool in the prevention of type 2 diabetes in obese children. "
http://care.diabetesjournals.org/content/28/5/1175.short

Further Reading

1. Chronic stress and obesity: A new view of "comfort food". http://www.pnas.org/content/100/20/11696.short
2. Chronic stress, glucocorticoids, insulin and obesity, Mary Dallman.
http://www.endocrine-abstracts.org/ea/0019/ea0019s10.htm
3. Magnesium Deficiency Is Associated With Insulin Resistance in Obese Children, Milagros di Huerta, MD et al.
http://care.diabetesjournals.org/content/28/5/1175.short

Module 6 - Magnesium - the Ultimate Energy Mineral

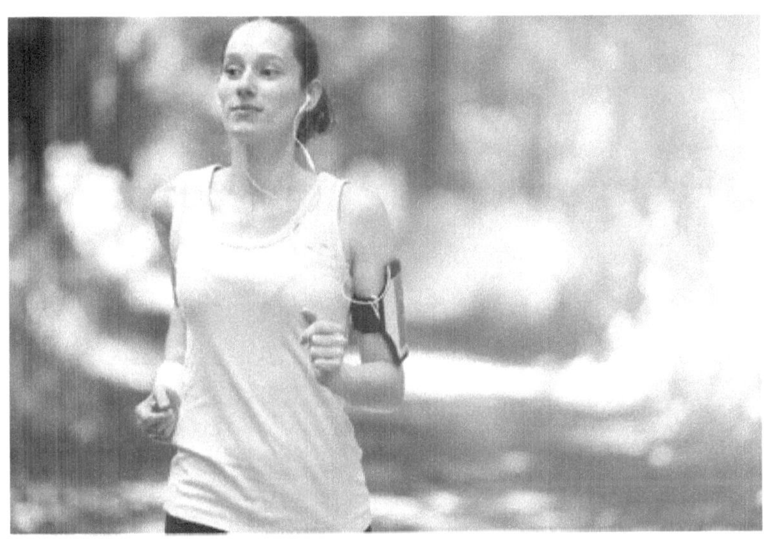

Unit 1 – Magnesium - the Energy Mineral

Magnesium is the ultimate 'energy' mineral. Without magnesium energy simply cannot be produced. This is because magnesium is required in the production of energy-rich bonds and the release of energy within the cell, from ATP - the "energy" molecule of each cell. If ATP is not bound by magnesium, then the cell simply cannot survive. Fatigue often responds well to magnesium supplementation.

Researchers with the USDA Agricultural Research Service recruited 10 postmenopausal women to participate in a three-phase diet and exercise study. During phase one (35 days), the women followed a controlled diet that delivered an adequate amount of magnesium. The current Recommended Dietary Allowance (RDA) for women is 320 mg daily. For men; 420 mg daily.

In the second phase (93 days), each subject consumed a diet that contained less than half the RDA for magnesium. In the final phase (49 days) the subjects returned to a diet with adequate magnesium. At the end of each phase, subjects took exercise tests, as well as physiological and biochemical tests.

Results showed that when magnesium intake was low, exercise increased heart rate and required more oxygen compared to exercising when magnesium intake was adequate. Also, when magnesium levels in muscles were low, more energy was required and subjects were tired more easily compared to subjects with adequate magnesium levels.

The crucial role of magnesium in energy production is a very important factor in the detoxification of all the body systems since effective detox requires energy, and without magnesium it becomes impossible. We will talk about it in more detail in the next unit.

Unit 2 – Metabolic Syndrome & Magnesium

Metabolic syndrome is a name for a combination of risk factors which occur together and increase the risk of diabetes mellitus, coronary heart disease, hypertension & stroke. The term first appeared in the 1950s to describe several symptoms connected with diabetes.

Metabolic syndrome is becoming more and more common worldwide, as the obesity rate is increasing not only in the Western world but also in Asia, Africa & South America.

The main reasons for the metabolic syndrome are ever-expanding waistlines through over-eating, a diet loaded with sugar and fatty foods, and a sedentary lifestyle. Other factors include genetic predisposition, hormonal changes associated with ageing, and high levels of stress.

Researchers in Taiwan have recently found that elderly people who were deficient in magnesium and whose intake of dietary magnesium was low, had the metabolic syndrome.

Consistent supplementation tops up magnesium levels in the body and helps correct abnormalities in the blood sugar levels, insulin resistance and levels of "bad" cholesterol. Adequate magnesium supplementation also helps to correct hormonal imbalances, which leads to rebalancing the body.

Magnesium works in tandem with calcium within the body, and when magnesium is deficient, excessive calcium escapes into the tissues, forming ossifications which lead to body rigidity and joint problems. It also takes part in the formation of atheromas which lead to blood vessel congestion called atherosclerosis.

Magnesium works as a natural cleanser for the body, collecting calcium from atheromas and ossified tissues. This results in the reversal of the symptoms of ageing, a general increase in energy levels, flexibility in the body and joint tissues. Magnesium supplementation also helps normalise blood pressure and sugar levels.

Natural ways of dealing with metabolic syndrome include:

- Dietary changes - exclude high sugar and high cholesterol food, alcohol, soft drinks, foods high in additives and artificial sweeteners.
- Introduce foods high in magnesium - leafy vegetables, nuts, pulses, brown rice, buckwheat, vegetables, seafood.
- Exercise - 1 hour a day is recommended.
- Oral magnesium supplementation.

- Transdermal magnesium supplementation - magnesium chloride oil sprayed or massaged over the body daily, Epsom salt baths, magnesium chloride baths.
- Vitamin D supplementation.
- Relaxation routine - choose an activity which makes you relaxed, and introduce it into your daily routine. It can be a sport, or a hobby, or simply having a chat with friends.

Unit 3 - Magnesium & Chronic Fatigue Syndrome

Two studies suggest that there is a possible organic explanation for chronic fatigue. British scientists report that low levels of magnesium may play a part in this illness with an unknown cause.

Although it is unclear whether magnesium injections reported improvements in their condition. The findings were published in the March 30 issue of "The Lancet" a renowned British medical journal.

The studies were conducted by Dr Michael J. Campbell, a medical statistician at Southampton General Hospital. Ivan M. Cox, a medical student at the University of Southampton and Dr David Dowson, a Southampton physician.

"This study shows a dramatic improvement in a small group of people with this illness, but it is too soon to say that this is an appropriate treatment that will be of help to the vast majority of patients," said Dr. Jay A. Levy, a professor of Medicine at the University of California at San Francisco, who has been searching for a possible viral cause of the disease.

Chronic fatigue patients usually complain about malaise lasting several months or years and nonspecific flu-like symptoms, including headaches, fever and muscle pain. They also suffer from an inability to think clearly, irritability and depression.

The researchers said they had decided to explore magnesium levels in patients with chronic fatigue because malabsorption of magnesium had been associated with lethargy and weakness. They did a case study and found that 20 patients suffering from chronic fatigue had slightly lower red-cell magnesium concentrations than did 20 healthy subjects matched for age, sex and social class.

In a clinical trial involving 32 patients with chronic fatigue syndrome, 15 patients were randomly given intramuscular injections of magnesium sulfate every week for six weeks and 17 were given shots of water.

The patients were not aware of which treatment they were receiving. Before and after the treatment, patients completed a questionnaire asking about their energy levels, pain, perception, sleep patterns, sense of social isolation, emotional reactions and physical mobility.

Twelve of the 15 patients treated with the magnesium said they had benefited and reported higher energy levels, better emotional states and less pain: just three patients who received the dummy shots claimed any improvement.

Yet to be determined is why magnesium levels were so low in these patients and if this is the case in the majority of chronic fatigue patients. Doctors have only recently started to take chronic fatigue syndrome seriously after years of dismissing it as little more than a figment of a patient's imagination." http://www.mgwater.com/chroniclz.shtml

Module 7 - Magnesium for Heavy Metals and Radiation Detox

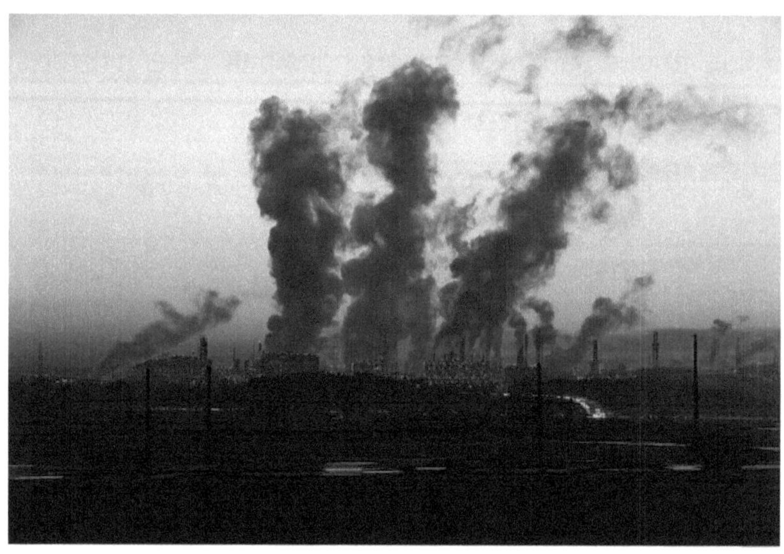

Unit 1 – Role of Magnesium in Detox - General Information

Magnesium plays a very important role in detoxification, in many ways:

- It provides the energy needed for detox by activating the energy-producing ATP-molecule. Without magnesium, energy cannot be produced, so detoxification is not possible.
- It stimulates the sodium-potassium exchange on the cell wall which regulates the potassium level inside and outside the cell thus stimulating the cell cleansing.
- Magnesium regulates the calcium content inside the cell preventing cellular calcification and premature ageing.
- Magnesium protects the cell against oxidation and damage by free radicals.
- Magnesium protects the body from heavy metals such as cadmium, lead, nickel, aluminium, mercury.
- Magnesium is crucial to protecting the brain against damage by heavy metals.

To keep the body free from toxins, it is vital to maintain optimal magnesium levels. There are several ways in which it can be achieved:

1. Magnesium-rich diet

2. Oral supplementation with magnesium

3. Transdermal Magnesium Therapy.

Unit 2 - Magnesium for Heavy Metal and Radiation Detox

Heavy metals

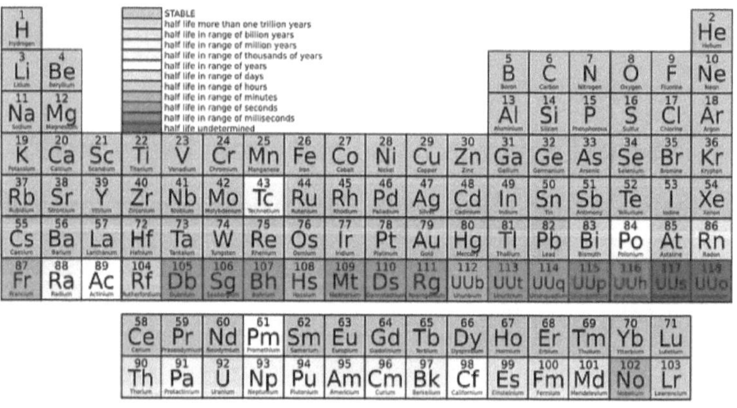

There is a debate as to what constitutes a heavy metal.

Some use the atomic weight (heavy for heavy metals),

while others base the name of the element valency (ability to bind other chemical elements, which is high for heavy metals).

The majority of researchers who write about heavy metal toxicity define any metal which is dangerous to human health in small amounts. Heavy metal toxicity can arise from acute or prolonged exposure to certain substances which contain heavy metals.

Many of the elements that can be considered heavy metals have no known benefit to humans. Such elements include lead, mercury, arsenic and cadmium. However, other metals are essential to human biochemical processes.

For example, zinc takes part in various enzymatic reactions, vitamin B-12 includes cobalt as part of it, and haemoglobin contains iron. Copper, manganese, selenium, chromium, and molybdenum are all trace elements, which play an important role in the human body. Other metals are used therapeutically in medicine. They include aluminium, bismuth, gold, gallium, lithium, and silver. Any of these elements may damage the body if taken in excessive quantity or if the usual mechanisms of elimination are impaired.

Heavy metal toxicity may be caused by many factors. Symptoms vary according to the metal, the total dose absorbed, and whether the exposure is acute or chronic. The age of the person can also influence toxicity. For example, young children are more prone to the effects of lead exposure because they absorb several times the per cent ingested compared with adults and because their brain is still growing and developing, so has more plasticity. Even brief exposures may influence developmental processes.

The route of exposure is also important. Elemental mercury is relatively inert in the gastrointestinal tract and also poorly absorbed through intact skin. However, if inhaled or injected, elemental mercury may have disastrous effects.

Heavy metals affect the body in various ways. They can cause many symptoms, starting from mild discomfort, leading to more serious symptoms, such as vomiting, diarrhoea, loss of consciousness, mental retardation, chronic diseases, cancer, and even death. Many of the symptoms have been covered when describing the toxins. This table gives a short overview of the most common heavy metal toxicity symptoms - https://www.ncbi.nlm.nih.gov/pmc/articles/PMC3113373/

Radioactive metals

Here is how The Medical Dictionary defines radioactive metals: "an element subject to spontaneous degeneration of its nucleus accompanied by the emission of alpha particles, beta particles, or gamma rays. All elements with atomic numbers greater than 83 are radioactive. Naturally occurring radioactive elements include radium, thorium, and uranium. Several radioactive elements not found in nature have been produced by the bombardment of stable elements with subatomic particles in a cyclotron."

Radiation can result from human activities and natural sources. The human environment has always been radioactive and results in 85% of radiation a human body is exposed to. It includes cosmic radiation, radiation from earth and rocks, radioactive gas emitted by volcanic rocks, uranium ore, radon gas. In most cases it is safe, and we don't even notice its effects.

Radiation arising from human activities makes up to 15% of the public's exposure every year. This radiation is no different from natural radiation, except that it can be controlled. Much of it involves exposure to X-rays and other medical procedures. A very small percentage - less than 1% - is a result of testing of nuclear weapons and the generation of electricity at nuclear power plants.

Radiation is used in small doses in medicine - for cancer treatment and x-rays. It is when exposure is chronic or accidental that problems happen. Exposure can be external (not penetrating the body) and internal (when the radioactive material gets into the body via water, food and air). Internal radiation is deemed the most dangerous of the two.

The effects of radiation can be from mild to devastating - depending on the intensity and period of exposure. "The radiation causes cellular degradation due to damage to DNA and other key molecular structures within the cells in various tissues. This destruction, particularly because it affects the ability of cells to divide normally, in turn, causes the symptoms...

The onset and type of symptoms depend on radiation exposure. Relatively smaller doses result in gastrointestinal effects, such as nausea and vomiting, and symptoms related to falling blood counts, and predisposition to infection and bleeding. Relatively larger doses can result in neurological effects and rapid death. Treatment of acute radiation syndrome is generally supportive with blood transfusions and antibiotics, with some more aggressive treatments, such as bone marrow transfusions, being required in extreme cases.

Similar symptoms may appear months to years after exposure as the chronic radiation syndrome when the dose rate is too low to cause the acute form. Radiation exposure

can also increase the probability of developing some other diseases, mainly different types of cancers. These diseases are sometimes referred to as radiation sickness, but they are never included in the term acute radiation syndrome."
https://en.wikipedia.org/wiki/Acute_radiation_syndrome

How magnesium helps to detoxify the body from heavy metals and radiation

Minerals play a vital role not only in detoxification of the body from heavy metals. They also help protect body tissues from further radioactive damage. Popular thinking is that radiation protection mostly involves using iodine, while supplementation in such vital minerals as magnesium and selenium is being often overlooked.

Magnesium supports all the body systems and detoxification processes. It provides the body with the energy it needs to ensure the elimination of toxins. Magnesium is also an integral part of glutathione - a detoxifying agent which protects the body from oxidative damage. It binds toxins into soluble substances excreting them with urine through the kidneys.

When magnesium is deficient, the body cannot produce sufficient glutathione, leading to cellular damage from free radicals, which leaves them exposed to further radioactive damage. Liver, kidneys, the heart, the lungs, as well as other organs of the body all have glutathione, and with magnesium deficiency, all of these vital organs are exposed to radiation.

Dr Mark Sircus writes: "Just about everyone who is writing about protocols for radiation toxicity is forgetting about the importance of magnesium salts. Magnesium is a crucial factor in the natural self-cleansing and detoxification responses of the body. It stimulates the sodium-potassium pump on the cell wall and this initiates the cleansing process in part because the sodium-potassium-ATPase pump regulates intracellular and extracellular potassium levels.

Cell membranes contain a sodium/potassium ATPase, a protein that uses the energy of ATP to pump sodium ions out of the cell, and potassium ions into the cell. The pump works all of the time, like a bilge pump in a leaky boat, pumping K+ and Na+ in and out, respectively... Load up on magnesium oil, magnesium bath flakes, Dead Sea salt and Epsom Salts". http://publications.imva.info/

Of course, heavy metal and radioactive detox must include a whole range of measures and must be performed at a medical establishment. However, as a preventative and complementary measure, the use of magnesium salts and other minerals, such as clay and zeolite, play a very important role.

Module 8 - Magnesium - the Anti-ageing Mineral. Symptoms, Causes & Theories of Ageing. Can Magnesium Reverse Ageing?

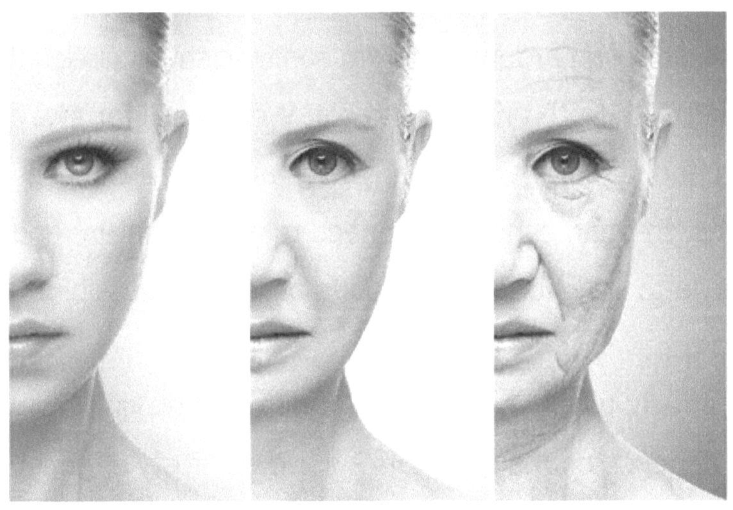

Unit 1 - Symptoms, Causes & Theories of Ageing

The idea of staying forever young has been occupying the human mind for thousands of years. People have been inventing all sorts of remedies to ward off the onset of age.

Nowadays scientists are looking into the genetic picture and how life and youth can be extended indefinitely based corrective adjustments to our genetic make-up.

There are even arguments from some scientific circles that ageing and death are preventable. We are still far away from finding out if there is any substance behind these claims. In the meantime, we need to rely on nature and our lifestyle to stay fit and look young as long as possible.

Age affects us all, even though in different ways. How we age depends on many factors - our diet, lifestyle, genetics, diet, social factors, financial circumstances, geolocation, demographics, genetics, a general state of health, the amount of stress we are exposed to, the environment and quite a lot of other factors. People of the same age may look different.

We can talk about the chronological, biological and social age of a person. Chronological age is the number of years the person has lived. Biological age shows the age the person feels and looks like, their health and their energy levels.

The social age is determined by the way the person perceives themselves, dresses, behaves, the circle of people they associate themselves with, their hobbies, pastimes and activities. It is also determined by how they are perceived in society.

Typical signs of ageing

- We become less physically active.
- Our skin becomes a lot less supple.
- Wrinkles and age spots appear on the face and body.
- The hair turns grey.
- Mobility becomes impaired, due to degenerative changes in the joints.
- Bones become a lot less dense.
- Hearing and vision become impaired.

- Our health becomes less strong, with the immune system becoming less efficient.
- Our response to challenging situations becomes less effective.
- We become heavier due to the accumulation of fat around the body.
- Our views, tastes and preferences change.
- Our behaviour changes.
- Our mental reaction and ability to learn new things slow down.
- Our dress sense changes.
- Our sex life becomes less exciting.
- Our hobbies, activities and pastimes change.

Having said that, this is not true for all. Some people change less than others. They stay young at heart, and it is reflected not only in how they look, behave, feel, or dress, but also how others see them as well. When a person's social and biological age remain in low figures, their life expectancy increases.

What determines how fast we age?

- Our genetic programming.
- The environment we live and work in.
- The climate we live in.
- Socio-economic factors. People living in deprivation are much more likely to age earlier.
- The amount and frequency of stress we are exposed to.
- Our general state of health.
- The food we eat.
- The water we drink.
- The air we breathe.
- The amount of time we work.
- The amount of time we sleep.
- The quality and quantity of breaks we have.
- The quality of our relationships.
- The people we associate with.
- Our general state of mind.
- Our spiritual pursuits.
- The quality of our sex life.
- General satisfaction with life.

- Creative pursuits we engage in.
- The way we look after ourselves.
- How active we are.
- Our will to remain young.

Some scientific theories on the subject of ageing

- **Evolutionary theory** - this theory argues that our lifespan, just like genotypes, is selected through evolutionary processes.
- **Accumulative waste theory** - we accumulate toxic waste over our lifetime, and this causes degeneration of the cells, leading to ageing.
- **"Wear and tear" theory** - argues that changes which happen as a result of ageing accumulate over time.
- **Error accumulation theory** - ageing results from chance events which gradually damage the genetic code.
- **Autoimmune theory** - ageing results from an increase in autoantibodies that attack the body's

tissues.

- **DNA damage theory** - this theory stipulates that ageing happens as a result of DNA damage over the lifetime. DNA damage is the most common cause of cancer, which is more common in older age.

Generally, ageing is a very complex process, and there is no single cause of it. There is also a train of thought that ageing may be an illness which can be treated. There is a lot of scientific research which proves that the lifespan can be extended. However, it may take some time to develop technologies which will allow for it, and we are not there yet. For this reason, our best bet is on taking every possible step to stay young naturally.

Further Reading

1. Why we age. - http://www.marquette.edu/magazine/recent.php?subaction=showfull&id=1281450540

2. Why do we age and is there anything we can do about it? - http://genetics.thetech.org/original_news/news10

3. Why do we age? A review of the theories of ageing - http://www.senescence.info/aging_theories.html

4. Magnesium Linked To Aging Mystery & Calcifications - http://www.mgwater.com/agingcal.shtml

Unit 2 - Can Magnesium Reverse Ageing?

In his book "Holy Water, Sacred Oil", Dr Norman Shealy documents about 90 health matters that are immediately related to magnesium deficiency. Also, Dr Shealy draws a strong correlation between magnesium levels and DHEA (dehydroepiandrosterone - a hormone produced by the adrenal glands which functions as a precursor to male and female sex hormones). He has also determined that when the body is presented with adequate levels of magnesium at the cellular level, the body will begin to naturally produce DHEA.

Since DHEA comprises the basic bio-marker for ageing, the long-term use of large doses of magnesium in an available form will significantly bring up DHEA levels and thus produce true **age reversal** results. Dr Shealy refers to DHEA as the master hormone. Adequate levels of DHEA cause the production of all of the other hormones.

The depletion of sex hormones is connected with a lot of symptoms of ageing. Stimulating a return to healthy and well-balanced levels of these hormones can give rise to a recovering of youthful energy. Indeed, through the application of magnesium oil, middle-aged women have described complete reprieve from menopausal symptoms and some have even returned to their menstrual cycle.

Dr Shealy has stated that once anyone starts regular use of magnesium oil, the ageing process has arrested and true age reversal has begun. As we have stopped ageing, time is no longer working against us. This institutes an unbelievable peace of mind and body.

Module 9 - Magnesium for a Healthy Heart

Unit 1 - Magnesium for a Healthy Heart & Circulation

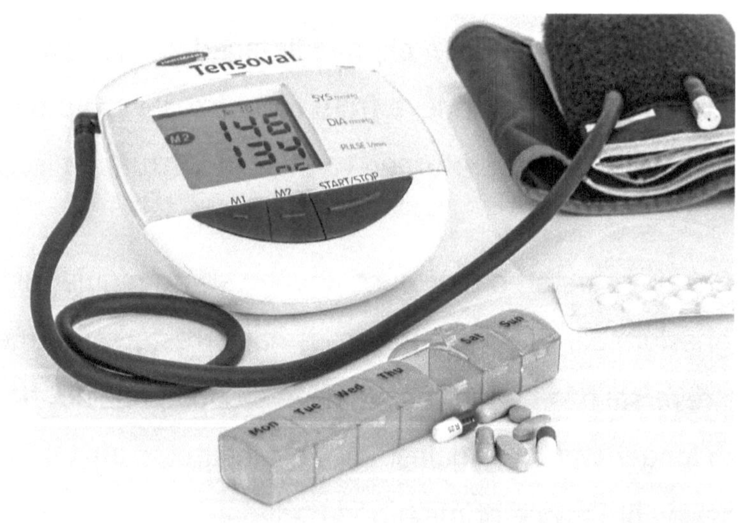

Magnesium is undoubtedly the most essential element in the prevention and treatment of heart disease and strokes. It has been established that people suffering from heart-related problems have very low magnesium and high calcium levels in their bodies.

High calcium levels and insufficient magnesium lead to a narrowing and hardening of arteries reducing their elasticity at the same time, which increases blood pressure and risk of heart attacks and strokes.

Atherosclerosis, the condition which involves calcium and cholesterol deposits in the arterial walls, is closely linked to magnesium deficiency. Not only does magnesium relax and dilate arteries and prevent the formation of scar tissue as a result of inflammations happening due to magnesium deficiency, but it also lowers cholesterol deposits by removing their major component, calcium, from the fatty plaques in the arterial walls, thus normalising blood pressure and reducing the risk of heart attacks and strokes.

There is extensive research showing that when patients with coronary heart disease are treated with high doses of magnesium injections, their survival rate increases dramatically.

Worldwide, intake of magnesium has decreased and that of calcium has increased - due to high use of food products (e.g. dairy) which are abundant in calcium and low in magnesium, sugary food and drinks, as well as the general depletion of soils of magnesium.

This, as well as other factors, such as unhealthy nutrition and lifestyles, high level of stress and lack of exercise, have resulted in an unprecedented increase in the number of people suffering from heart-related and circulatory problems.

Potassium (coming from fertilisers) is thought to be another culprit leading to magnesium-depleted soils and, as a result, a catastrophic reduction of magnesium in our diets.

Areas where the soil is low in calcium and potassium and high in magnesium, show a much lower rate of conditions connected with magnesium deficiency, and this, of course, includes heart disease.

In her article "MAGNESIUM IN ONCOGENESIS AND IN ANTI-CANCER TREATMENT: INTERACTION WITH MINERALS AND VITAMINS", Mildred S. Seelig, M.D., M.P.H. says about the risk of mortality from cardiovascular disease:

"Greater morbidity and mortality from cardiovascular disease is directly correlated with water softness and diet. Metabolic balance studies, with normal young adults on their usual diets, show that the lesser American Mg intake by adults, causing negative Mg balance, than in the Orient, correlates with the much higher death rate from ischemic heart disease (IHD) in the USA.

Most American diets provide less than 70% of the 1980 recommended dietary allowance (RDA) of Mg. Experimental and clinical studies and epidemiologic findings indicate that it is Mg, rather than Ca, that protects against IHD, myocardial infarcts and sudden unexpected cardiac death caused by arrhythmias."

http://www.mgwater.com/cancer.shtml

Positive results have been achieved in numerous studies aimed at regulating blood pressure with increased intake of magnesium. It works by relaxing the blood vessels which in turn expand, thus reducing the pressure of the flowing blood on arterial walls. This property has long been known to orthodox practitioners. The spasm-relieving property of magnesium is being routinely used in A&E departments to minimise the risks associated with the heart attack.

Dr Andrea Rosanoff, PhD, writes: "By 1957 low magnesium was shown to be, strongly, convincingly, a cause of atherogenesis and the calcification of soft tissues. But this research was widely and immediately ignored as cholesterol and the high saturated-fat diet became the culprits to fight. Ever since this early 'wrong turn', more and more peer-reviewed research has shown that low magnesium is associated with all known cardiovascular risk factors, such as cholesterol and high blood pressure."
http://www.medicalnewstoday.com/articles/255783.php

Magnesium and blood pressure

Being a natural relaxant, magnesium is needed to keep the blood vessels supple and open. It also regulates the amount of calcium and cholesterol in the blood. If the magnesium level is low, the blood starts circulating too much calcium and cholesterol - ideal materials for the plaque formation. Plus, insufficient magnesium leading too much calcium leads to inflammations and rigidity of the tissues, including blood vessels.

Inflammation can lead to damage to the blood vessels, which can result in the formation of scar tissue. An arterial plaque has more chances of forming in the area of scar tissue. Once a plaque is formed, it keeps growing, and eventually, the opening narrows down, so blood pressure goes up. It's like with a garden hose - try pinching or bending it to restrict the water flow and see what happens.

Further Reading

"Magnesium - the Ultimate Heart Medicine" e-book, Dr Mark Sircus - http://publications.imva.info/index.php/e-books/magnesium-the-ultimate-heart-medicine-e-book.html

Unit 2 - Magnesium, Potassium and Arrhythmia, Sheehan J P, Seelig M S (Study)

This is a very important article reflecting results of research into how magnesium and potassium deficiency brought about by the use of diuretics in patients with high blood pressure can lead to arrhythmia, cardiac infarction and even sudden death.

"Magnesium (Mg) and potassium (K) deficiencies frequently coexist in clinical practice, most commonly as a result of poor gastrointestinal absorption or renal conservation, secondary to intrinsic disease or its treatment. Suboptimal Mg intake makes its renal conservation critical, especially in seriously ill catabolic hospitalized patients, many of whom have protein-calorie-malnutrition, which further compromises cation homeostasis.

Prescription of diuretics and other agents that cause Mg- and K-wasting can readily provoke a loss of intracellular (i.c.) cations, that is not diagnosed by tests of serum levels. Direct i.c. measurements may disclose major deficiencies, that can exist in the presence of normal serum values. In the case of Mg, loading tests may provide indirect evidence of i.e. deficiency that can complicate the care of high-risk patients.

Mg deficiency disrupts cellular function and integrity, with impairment of cellular bioenergetics, increased membrane permeability, and dysfunction of the Na/K adenosine triphosphatase [ATP] pump and other enzyme systems, resulting in K-depletion and Ca-overload. K-therapy alone may fail to correct low serum and/or i.c. K-level. Indeed, the frequent use of high doses of K, without correction of the Mg deficiency, can further exacerbate the combined deficiencies, through stimulation of aldosterone secretion.

Deficiency of either Magnesium of K is arrhythmogenic: the aged ischemic myocardium in the setting of myocardial infarction is particularly vulnerable to the cation deficiencies. Refractory ventricular and atrial arrhythmias have responded to repletion of either or both cations, after a failure of conventional anti-arrhythmic agents that were given without correction of the deficiencies.

Increased cardiac mortality in mild hypertension trials... led to speculation as to arrhythmogenicity of the diuretic-associated hypokalemia as a risk factor for sudden death. Extracellular (e.c.) changes in K are more important in determining resting membrane potential and electrical stability of the heart than are the cardiac level – which may be preserved in the face of total body deficiency – provided there is not concomitant Mg depletion. Thus, complacency regarding total body K in the face of small changes reported in hypertensives treated with diuretics is unfounded, because of the critical roles of i.c. K and Mg – both of which can be depleted by long-term use of diuretics.

Catecholamine surges can also have profound adverse effects on e.c. K, through enhanced skeletal muscle K uptake. This can be especially critical in patients with myocardial infarction. Diuretic-induced intensification of Mg deficiency increases the vulnerability to arrhythmia of hypertensive patients, both through a direct effect on K, and by increasing the secretion of catecholamines - which in turn adversely influences myocardial Mg uptake, and induces lipolysis, which further reduces the available Mg pool. K is antiarrhythmic in patients with myocardial infarction in combination with glucose and insulin. It has been suggested that the addition of Mg... might improve the therapeutic effect "

http://www.mgwater.com/seelig_magnesium_potassium_and_arrhythmia.pdf

Unit 3 – The Link between Inflammation, Heart Disease & Magnesium (Scientific Studies)

Study 1

Dr Michael Eades has this to say about magnesium and inflammation:

The lipid hypothesis of heart disease is rapidly being supplanted by the inflammatory hypothesis, which, for my money, is much more on the mark. The researchers who have spent their careers doing cholesterol research are not going down without a fight, however. Whereas most of the speakers at medical conferences always used to show graphs demonstrating that as cholesterol levels went up, so did the risk for heart disease. Now most speakers are showing graphs demonstrating that elevated cholesterol in combination with an elevated C-reactive protein (a measure of inflammation) is a better gauge of heart disease risk. I predict that over the next few years, the cholesterol part of these graphs will slowly disappear.

As the inflammatory hypothesis becomes more accepted, more and more physicians will be checking C-reactive protein levels along with a few other inflammatory yardsticks to determine the inflammatory status of their patients. If the C-reactive protein level is found to be elevated, then steps can be taken, not just to reduce the C-reactive protein, but to treat the underlying inflammation so that the C-reactive protein a marker of this underlying inflammation will normalize.

https://proteinpower.com/drmike/2005/07/29/magnesium-and-inflammation/

Study 2

"Tuesday, November 24, 2009 - Byron Richards, CCN.
A new study of 3,713 postmenopausal women shows that magnesium is a powerful anti-inflammatory nutrient. Each 100 mg of magnesium per day was associated with a significant reduction in various inflammatory markers.

Magnesium is the most lacking mineral in the human diet. This is due primarily to Big Agribusiness farming practices that have stripped our soils of vital minerals needed for human health. It is complicated by processed diets lacking in magnesium-containing fresh fruits and vegetables. When you consider that inflammation is behind almost all health problems the consequence of eating a magnesium-deficient diet becomes obvious.

The study showed that inflammatory markers such as CRP (C-reactive protein), TNFa (tumour necrosis factor-alpha), and IL6 (interleukin 6) were all reduced when magnesium intake was higher. These are common inflammatory markers that are often elevated with the diseases of ageing.

Furthermore, various inflammatory markers relating to the walls of arteries were also reduced when magnesium was adequate. Inflammation on the lining of the arteries is required for plaque formation. Reducing such inflammation is highly protective of arterial health.

It is not a stretch to say that if public health officials did nothing other than ensuring vitamin D and magnesium sufficiency the entire health of a nation would be drastically improved and health care costs would be significantly lower."

http://www.wellnessresources.com/health/articles/magnesium_the_anti-inflammatory_mineral/

Module 10 - Magnesium for Healthy Immunity and Cancer Prevention

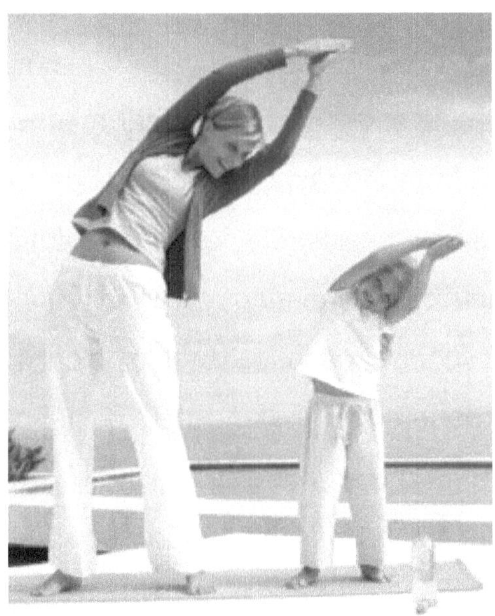

Unit 1 - The Link between Magnesium and Immunity

As the 2nd most abundant mineral in the human body,

magnesium plays a very important part of our body's response to infection. Here is an abstract from a study published in the European Journal of Clinical Nutrition:

"Regarding the relation between Mg and the immune system, several groups leading in Nutrition and Immunology have shown evidence that magnesium plays a key role in the immune response; that is, as a co-factor for immunoglobulin synthesis, C'3 convertase, immune cell adherence, antibody-dependent cytolysis, IgM lymphocyte binding, macrophage response to lymphokines and T helper–B cell adherence (Galland, 1988)." ("Possible roles of magnesium on the immune system", M Tam, S Gómez, M González-Gross and A Marcos, European Journal of Clinical Nutrition (2003) 57, 1193–1197. doi:10.1038/sj.ejcn.1601689).

Dr Mark Sircus observes in his book "Transdermal Magnesium Therapy": "Our bodies are best served when they are brimming with magnesium reserves and we need to absorb a sufficient amount every day. A magnesium saturated body will have a tougher immune system that will

fight more easily against infections and influenza."
("Transdermal Magnesium Therapy", 2007, p.200).

Here is an abstract from another study which shows a correlation between magnesium and immunity:
"Hypomagnesemia [magnesium deficiency] promotes low-grade inflammation as demonstrated by elevated concentrations of C-Reactive Protein (CRP) and TNF-α [10,11]. Low Mg is independently associated with elevated hsCRP levels [11,12]. Subjects who consume less than 75% of RDA were 1.94 times more likely to have elevated serum CRP levels than consuming above the RDA [13] and, in another study, the number of subjects with CRP > 3 mg. L-1 significantly decreased from the lowest to the highest tertile of dietary Mg [14]. Adults who consumed less than the Mg RDA were 1.48-1.75times more likely to have elevated CRP than adults who consumed more than the RDA [7]. Additionally, low Mg induces increases in circulating substance P that stimulates systemic inflammatory stress [15,16].

Various mechanisms may explain the role of Mg in modulating immune function. Mg potentiates iron–transferrin binding, an important contribution to offsetting oxidative stress [17]. *Mg reduces oxidative stress through stabilization of DNA.* [18].

Unit 2 - Magnesium for Cancer Prevention

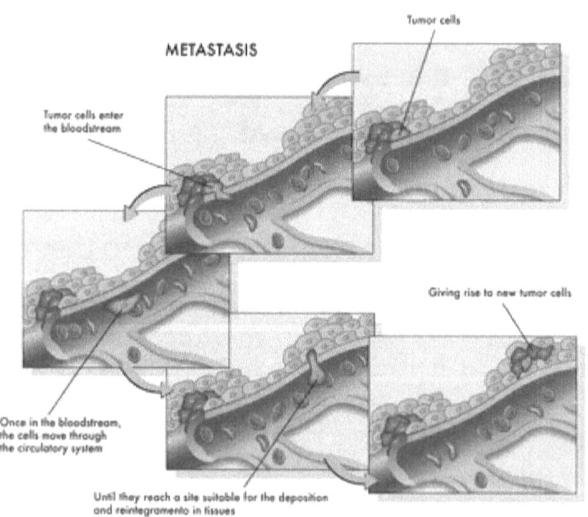

It is hard to overestimate how important magnesium is not only in prevention but also in the treatment of cancer.

Various studies have shown that magnesium-poor diet which includes mostly processed, sugary and fatty food and deficiency of magnesium in soil result in higher incidences of cancer among the population.

On May 19, 1931, Dr Schrumpf-Pierron presented a paper entitled "On the Cause of the Rarity of Cancer in Egypt". In it he wrote:

"(1) Cancer for Egypt is about one-tenth that of Europe and America.

(2) In Egypt, cancer is less frequent in-country fellahin than in the Egyptians who live in the towns and who have adopted Europeanized dietary habits.

(3) The degree of malignancy of Egyptian cancers is less than that of European cancers. They develop less quickly and have less of a tendency to invade neighbouring tissues.

(4) The type of cancer which is the most frequent in all the countries rich in cancer is a cancer of the digestive tract, which represents 40 to 50 per cent of all cancers. In the case of Egyptians, this type of cancer is remarkably rare; in the country fellahin, practically nonexistent".

http://www.mgwater.com/rod02.shtml

He concluded that the prevalence of potassium in the soils of European countries with low levels of magnesium result in an increased risk of cancer among the population. In Egypt, both the soil and diet are rich in magnesium, and for this reason, he saw it as the main factor in the very low cancer rate among Egyptians.

"An intoxication of potash - an excess of potash poisons - can "kill" the soil where the food is grown. It poisons the plants, then man. Besides, several other authorities have already accused potash of producing cancer. Theis and Benedikt, as will as Mentrier, have already stated that the higher amount of potash in cancerous tissue, which is a radioactive body, would cause the multiplication of cancerous cells". http://www.mgwater.com/rod02.shtml

In her article "MAGNESIUM IN ONCOGENESIS AND IN ANTI-CANCER TREATMENT: INTERACTION WITH MINERALS AND VITAMINS", Mildred S. Seelig, M.D., M.P.H. says that magnesium deficiency can both decrease and paradoxically protect against cancer. For example, magnesium supplementation of those who are magnesium-deficient (e.g. chronic alcoholics) may protect them against developing some tumours.

"Optimal Mg intake may be prophylactic against the initiation of some neoplasms." The author then points out the correlation between water hardness/softness and longevity: "Since environmental factors have been judged likely to contribute to most human cancers, it is worth effort to ascertain if there are protective geochemical agents. Determining what it is in different geographic regions, that affects life expectancy, provides one approach. The largest area in the United States of America (USA) with increased longevity is in the north and central plains; the largest area with decreased longevity is in the south-eastern coastal area. These are hard and soft water regions, respectively".

Worldwide studies have established a **reverse correlation of magnesium deficiency in soil and prevalence of certain types of cancer.** "A Russian report showed that stomach cancer is four times more common (40/100,000) in Ukraine where the Mg content of soil and drinking water is low than it is in Armenia (10/100,000) where the Mg content is more than twice as high. (14,66-68) A more recent morphologic and statistical analysis of neoplastic deaths in two Polish communities(69) disclosed a nearly three-fold higher death rate in the one in a low soil Mg area (27%) than in the one with high soil Mg (10%).

The malignancies accounting for the differences were mainly adeno- and squamous cell carcinomas in the gastrointestinal tract (61.3%) and respiratory system (22.3%)". "Correlation of high rates of leukaemia with low levels of Mg in soil and water is concordant with experiments showing that chronic Mg deficiency can cause lymphosarcomas and leukaemia in rats".

"Connective tissue, made up of fibroblastic cells that produced collagen type III, proliferated in the intestines of rats maintained on severely Mg-deficient diets for at least 8 weeks. A less Mg-restricted diet did not evoke such tumors." http://www.mgwater.com/cancer.shtml

"It is known that carcinogenesis induces magnesium distribution disturbances, causing magnesium mobilization through blood cells and magnesium depletion in non-neoplastic tissues. **Magnesium deficiency seems to be carcinogenic, and in the case of solid tumors, a high level of supplemented magnesium inhibits carcinogenesis.**[10] Both carcinogenesis and magnesium deficiency increase the plasma membrane permeability and fluidity. Scientists have found out that there is much less Mg++ binding to membrane phospholipids of cancer cells than to normal cell membranes.[11]

It has been suggested that magnesium deficiency may trigger carcinogenesis by increasing membrane permeability.[12] The membranes of magnesium-deficient cells seem to have a smoother surface and decreased membrane viscosity than normal cells, analogous to changes in human leukemia cells.[13],[14] And we find that lead (Pb) salts are more leukemogenic when given to magnesium-deficient rats than when they are given to magnesium-adequate rats, suggesting that magnesium is protective.[15]"

"Researchers from Japan's National Cancer Center in Tokyo have found that an increased intake of magnesium reduces a man's risk of colon cancer by over 50 percent. Men with the highest average intakes of magnesium (at least 327 mg/d) were associated with a 52 percent lower risk of colon cancer, compared to men who consumed the lowest average intakes. Published in the *Journal of Nutrition*,[2] the research studied 87,117 people with an average age of 57 and followed them for about eight years. Dietary intakes were assessed using a food frequency questionnaire. Average intakes of magnesium for men and women were 284 and 279 milligrams per day."

http://drsircus.com/medicine/magnesium-is-basic-to-cancer-treatment#_edn15

For cancer patients, regular magnesium supplementation becomes a matter of urgency and necessity, not simply a choice. **Dr Mark Sircus** recommends taking both oral magnesium supplements and using magnesium chloride transdermally, on the skin, in addition to other treatments. But of course, medical advice will need to be sought by any cancer patient before any supplementation, to avoid any clashes with the medication already being taken.

Module 11 - Magnesium for Healthy Liver and Kidneys

Unit 1 - Magnesium for Healthy Liver & Bile Flow

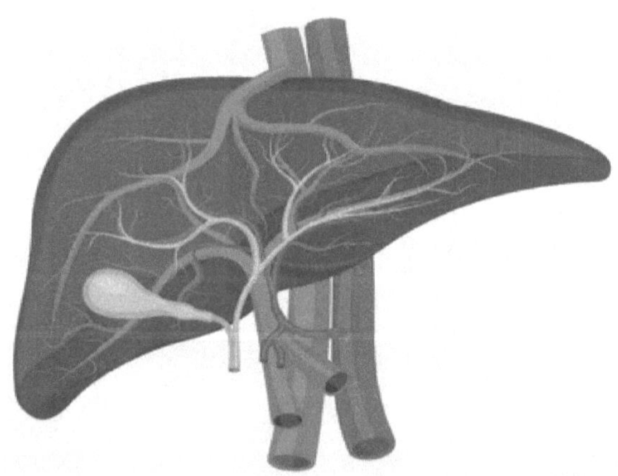

Liver - its role in detoxification

The liver is the main detoxification organ in the body, alongside the skin and kidneys, neutralising toxins produced internally as a result of metabolic processes, as well as external toxins - harmful organisms, products of pollution, heavy metals, toxins we get from food, drink, cigarettes, alcohol, drugs, air, things we buy, domestic chemicals, personal care products, medicines, etc.

The liver performs hundreds of tasks every minute, constantly synthesising, removing harmful substances, filtering, processing. The liver is involved in all systems of the body, including blood circulation, endocrine, digestive, nervous, immune, reproductive, eliminatory systems. It produces multiple enzymes and hormones which are required for various body processes.

The liver detoxifies the body in a complex series of chemical reactions. Many of the toxins circulating in the body as a result of metabolic activity are fat-soluble. One of the functions of the liver is to convert these fat-soluble substances into water-soluble ones so that they can be excreted from the body with bile or urine.

If the liver is not functioning properly, then it is unable to remove fat-soluble toxins efficiently, so they get deposited in the fatty tissues in the body and can stay there for years. So, the excess fat we carry contains a lot of fat-soluble toxic waste which keeps accumulating, leading to poor immunity, chronic fatigue, slow metabolism, weight gain, depression and other serious problems.

The liver is involved in the regulation of hormones in the body, constantly synthesising and breaking them down. If the liver is inefficient due to being overloaded with toxins, then this synthesis and elimination of unwanted hormones are compromised. This means that the hormones which the body no longer needs are not broken down and are accumulating in the body, mainly in the fatty tissues.

A good example is an excess oestrogen in women which gets deposited in fatty tissues causing all sorts of problems, such as heavy bleeding, weight gain, fibroids, development of tumours, etc.

Apart from what has been mentioned already, the liver is the powerhouse in the body, producing the energy in a long chain of enzymatic reactions, as a result of carbohydrate, fat and protein metabolism. Again, if its function is deficient, then the amount of energy it produces is insufficient for the body processes, resulting in slowing down of the whole body. On the whole, the liver determines how healthy a person feels. This is why naturopaths, first of all, examine the liver to check its efficiency and overall health.

What part does magnesium play in all this?

Magnesium is one of the most important and abundant minerals in the body. It is the main component in over 300 reactions. The liver uses a lot of magnesium since it is the nutrient processing, detoxifying and energy-producing "factory" in the body. Without magnesium, these processes would not take place.

Magnesium can become depleted as a result of an illness, alcohol abuse, insufficient magnesium in the diet, stress, physical exertion. Here is a result of a study of how liver magnesium is affected by alcohol abuse for example:

"The acute ingestion of alcohol causes a prompt, short-term increase in urinary excretion of magnesium. There are wide individual variations in the extent of this effect both in normal subjects and in chronic alcoholics. Patients who are already magnesium-depleted tend to lose less magnesium in response to alcohol intake.
http://findarticles.com/p/articles/mi_m0887/is_n10_v13/ai_15882994

What magnesium does for detox

1. It provides the energy needed for detox by activating the energy-producing ATP-molecule. Without magnesium, energy cannot be produced, so detoxification is not possible.
2. It stimulates the sodium-potassium exchange on the cell wall which regulates potassium level inside and outside the cell thus stimulating the cell cleansing.

3. Magnesium regulates calcium content inside the cell preventing cellular calcification and premature ageing.
4. Magnesium protects the cell against oxidation and damage by free radicals.
5. Magnesium protects the body from heavy metals such as cadmium, lead, nickel, aluminium, mercury.
6. Magnesium is crucial at protecting the brain against damage by heavy metals.

To keep the body free from toxins, it is vital to maintain optimal magnesium levels. There are several ways in which it can be achieved:

1. Magnesium-rich diet
2. Oral supplementation with magnesium
3. Transdermal magnesium therapy.

Transdermal magnesium therapy is one of the most effective ways to replenish magnesium in the body quickly and safely. This can be achieved in several ways described in this book.

Unit 2 - Kidney Stones & Magnesium

Kidney stones are quite common in the general population. Many of us do not even know we have them, due to their very small size. Much of the time they pass through the system unnoticed. It is when they grow to larger sizes and the kidneys try to expel them that they get trapped in the ureters, causing major problems - including excruciating pain.

"Risk factors include high urine calcium levels, obesity, certain foods, some medications, calcium supplements, hyperparathyroidism, gout and not drinking enough fluids. Stones form in the kidney when minerals in urine are at high concentration."
https://en.wikipedia.org/wiki/Kidney_stone_disease

Most kidney stones are formed in the presence of calcium and can include calcium oxalate, calcium phosphate or uric acid. The first two are responsible for most kidney stones, while uric acid forms only a relatively small percentage.

Possible causes for kidney stone formation

1. Acidic body environment due to a diet high in sugars, meat, alcohol & coffee. These acid-forming foods deplete the bones of calcium excreting it through the kidneys.
2. Calcium supplementation without sufficient magnesium in the diet can cause calcium overload in the body.
3. Dehydration causes the urine to become more concentrated which means it contains more calcium.
4. Soft drinks such as cola and others containing phosphoric acid. These also bind with bone calcium taking out of the body and getting deposited in the kidneys in the process.

The calcium-magnesium imbalance is the major factor in kidney stone formation. The main role of magnesium is to keep calcium in an ionic form to prevent it from forming crystals. It works even when we are dehydrated. However, when the levels of calcium and magnesium in the body are out of balance then excess calcium gets deposited in the body tissues and organs leading to calcification of the tissues and a formation of kidney stones.

Also, calcium crystal deposition in the tissues leads to all sorts of medical problems, such as osteoarthritis, gout, fibrositis, atherosclerosis, muscle spasms, etc.

Regular supplementation with magnesium corrects the calcium-magnesium imbalance in the body leading to the elimination of excess calcium from the kidneys and other body tissues and prevention of further kidney stone formation.

Dietary requirements to prevent the formation of kidney stones

- Increasing fluid intake to more than 2 litres per day (of total urine output)
- Increasing citric acid intake (lemons are the best

source)
- Reducing calcium supplementation
- Reducing products containing oxalic acid (peanuts, pecan nuts, cashew nuts, beets, rhubarb, wheat bran & chocolate) for people who are at a higher risk of forming kidney stones)
- Limiting the amount of salt in the food
- Moderate supplementation with vitamin C
- Reducing the intake of acid-forming food: meat and other animal protein, refined carbohydrates, cola and soft drinks.
- Introducing alkalising food into the diet.

If choosing oral supplementation with calcium and magnesium, the citrate form is best. "Sufficient dietary intake of magnesium and citrate inhibits the formation of calcium oxalate and calcium phosphate stones; also, magnesium and citrate operate synergistically to inhibit kidney stones. Magnesium's efficacy in subduing stone formation and growth is dose-dependent."

https://en.wikipedia.org/wiki/Kidney_stone_disease

Caution: people suffering from renal deficiency or any other kidney problems must always consult a medical practitioner before any supplementation is considered.

Module 12 - Magnesium for Allergies and Asthma

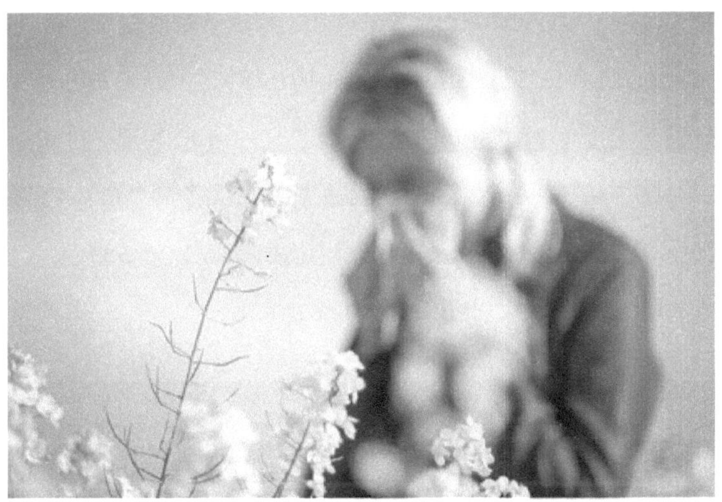

Unit 1 - Allergies, Food Intolerances and Magnesium

Allergic reactions are a very complex subject since it covers quite a lot of areas, such as a reaction to food and drinks, things we get in contact with (e.g. plants, chemicals), airborne particles, as well as medicines.

To sum it up, an allergic reaction is caused by the inability of the body to recognise a substance and reject as foreign. This causes several responses in the body, such as a release of IgE (Immunoglobulin E) - an antibody which is specific to that allergen. IgE attaches itself to mast cells - the cells found in the superficial tissues which are responsible for the release of histamine.

The next time we get into contact with the same allergen, mast cells start mobilising themselves to defend the body, releasing a whole number of chemicals, including histamine and prostaglandins.

Histamine release can cause the airways to constrict which brings about asthma-like symptoms. It can also make the blood vessels more permeable, which can lead to rashes and hives. Itchy eyes, sore throat, rashes and sneezing are just some signs of an allergic reaction. Sometimes only some symptoms show, and not others.

Hay fever is the most common form of allergy, but there are others too, such as the hives. Of course, we are not talking about much more complex and dangerous reactions, such as the nut allergy, or allergic reactions to certain medicines. These conditions must always be monitored by medical professionals.

In most cases what we call 'allergies', especially related to food, should be referred to as 'intolerances' or 'food sensitivities'. There is also another form of allergy called the 'autoimmune disease' when the body starts rejecting its tissues. However, it is a complex subject which deserves special coverage.

"In the book Encyclopedia of Natural Medicine, the authors note that food allergies are usually associated with low hydrochloric acid levels and poor digestion. The authors' rationale for this is that low stomach acid leaves food undigested and fermenting in the intestinal tract. This fermentation causes gas, bloating and stomach upset, the symptoms of irritable bowel syndrome. Undigested and fermented food causes the body to raise histamine levels, which produce allergic reactions. This is why people take antihistamines for allergies, to lower histamine levels. Interestingly, Mg is needed to reduce histamine levels.

Low stomach acid levels reduce levels of beneficial intestinal bacteria which is needed for absorption of magnesium... Mg deficiency has been implicated in allergies and allergic skin reaction in many studies on humans... Variations of allergies, skin allergies, and raised white blood cells have all been noted as features of many chronic disorders.

People with chemical sensitivities also commonly have other conditions linked to Mg deficits such as allergies, fibromyalgia, mitral valve prolapse and anxiety disorders. They also tend to have the temporomandibular joint disorder (TMJ), which has been linked to abnormalities of hyaluronic acid. Perhaps not coincidentally, hyaluronic acid is dependent upon magnesium for its synthesis. "

http://allergiessos.blogspot.co.uk/2011/02/allergy-control-mineral-supplementation.html

Unit 2 - Asthma and Magnesium – Studies

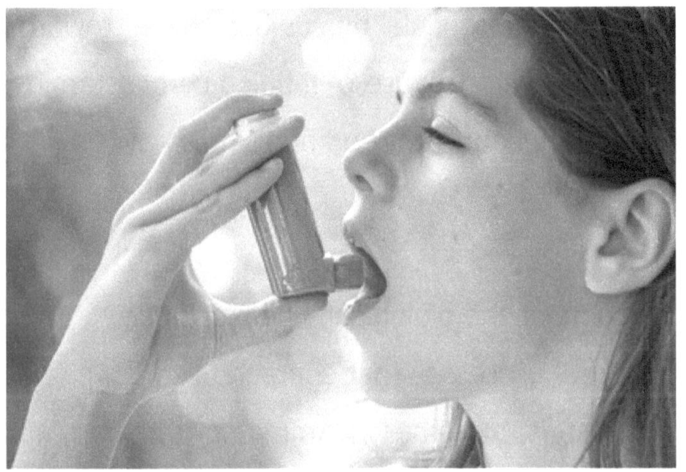

Asthma has been linked to Mg deficiency in a wide variety of studies. Results of two such studies are described below.

Study 1

Transdermal Magnesium Therapy Course for Clinic & Home Use

Harari M, Barzillai R, Shani J.

The recognition of asthma as an inflammatory disease has led over the past 20 years to a major shift in its pharmacotherapy. The previous emphasis on using relatively short-acting agents for relieving bronchospasms and for removing bronchial mucus has shifted toward long-term strategies with the use of inhaled corticosteroids, which successfully prevent and abolish airway inflammation.

Because some of the biological, chemical, and immunological processes that characterize asthma also underlie arthritis and other inflammatory diseases, and because many of these conditions have been successfully treated for the past 40 years at the Dead Sea, we were not surprised to realize and record the significant improvement in the asthmatic condition after a 4-week stay at the Dead Sea: lung function was improved, the number and severity of attacks were reduced, and the efficacy of beta2-agonist treatments was improved.

After reviewing the acute and chronic treatments of asthma in the clinic (including emergency rooms) with magnesium compounds, and the use of such salts as supplementary agents in respiratory diseases, we suggest that the improvement in the asthmatic condition at the Dead Sea may be due to absorption of this element through the skin and via the lungs, and due to its involvement in anti-inflammatory and vasodilatory processes".

https://www.ncbi.nlm.nih.gov/pubmed/9777879?dopt=Abstract

Study 2

Dr John Briffa says:

"Magnesium therapy was tried in a study published recently in the Journal of Asthma [1]. In it, 55 adults with mild-moderate asthma were treated with magnesium (170 mg, twice a day) or placebo over 6.5 months. Individuals had their lung function tested using peak expiratory flow (the maximum speed air can be expelled from the lungs) as well as something known as the methacholine challenge test.

Methacholine causes constriction of airways. In this test, subjects breath in methacholine and the dose of this drug required to induce constriction in the airways. The higher the dose of methacholine required, the less 'reactive' the airways would be judged to be.

Compared to those taking the placebo, those taking magnesium saw significant improvement in both their peak expiratory flow rate and methacholine challenge results".
http://www.drbriffa.com/blog/2010/01/29/magnesium-therapy-found-to-benefit-asthmatics/

Module 13 - Reproductive Health and Magnesium

Unit 1 - Reproductive Health and Magnesium

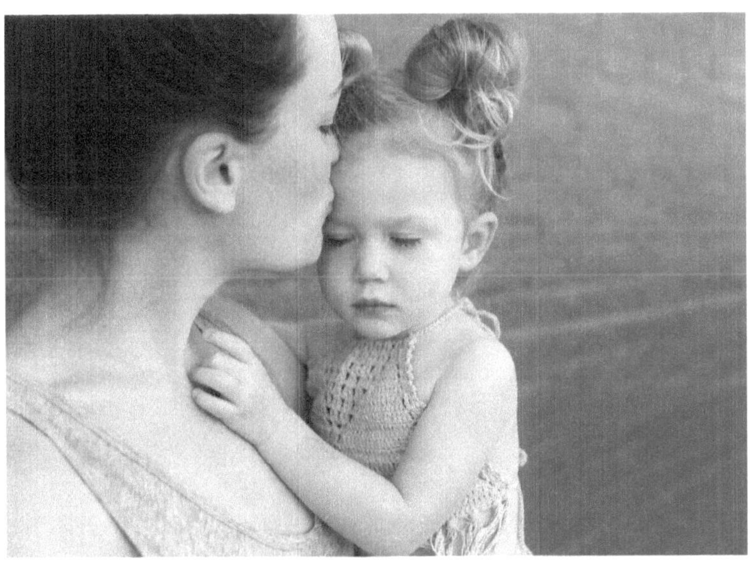

In this unit, we will look at a study of the correlation

between magnesium and sexuality as described by Dr Mark Sircus in his book "Transdermal Magnesium Therapy", 2007.

Taking part in over 300 chemical reactions, magnesium affects all the body systems. The health of the reproductive system is closely linked to magnesium levels in the body, both in men and women. Sexual drive and functions are hormone-dependent, and magnesium is a major element necessary for the production of all hormones.

Magnesium is crucial in the production of healthy sperm and eggs, as well as in all the reproductive processes - ovulation, conception, gestation, birth, lactation, establishing of a bond between mother and baby, healthy sexual relationships. "Sex, in particular, has become a major source of anxiety and stress for many of us and this is not all our fault... Magnesium is necessary for normal sexual functioning, yet is glossed over in its importance in nervous and endocrine function necessary for good sexual performance". (Mark Sircus, Transdermal Magnesium Therapy, 2007, p.234).

Magnesium levels are very high in the semen - higher than in the blood serum. Infertile men have been found to have half the level of magnesium in their semen as fertile men. " (Mark Sircus, Transdermal Magnesium Therapy, 2007, p.235)

Magnesium affects the production and transmission of all hormones in the body - serotonin, thyroid, estrogen, testosterone, insulin, neurotransmitters, etc. In his book, Dr Sircus plays special attention to the role of magnesium in the production of DHEA - dehydroepiandrosterone which "appears to protect every part of the body against the ravages of ageing" and is "flaunted as a "fountain of youth" (Mark Sircus, Transdermal Magnesium Therapy, 2007p.237, 241).

DHEA is a steroid hormone produced by the adrenal glands both in men and women. Its levels peak in puberty and drop in the early 30s. It is converted in the body into some hormones, including estrogen and testosterone, and affects muscle growth, libido, sperm production, and much more.

The publicity of the age-defying effect of DHEA on the body has led to a surge in the population taking it as a synthetic supplement says Dr Sircus, purchased both on prescription and over the counter. He points out a number of adverse effects resulting from such supplementation, including unwanted hair in women, acne, increased risk of ovarian cancer, breast cancer, prostate cancer in men, heart attacks).

At the same time, Dr Sircus points out that deficiency in DHEA leads not simply to ageing on all levels, but also "chronic inflammation, immune dysfunction, depression, rheumatoid arthritis, type 2 diabetes, greater risk of certain cancers, excess body fat, cognitive decline, heart disease in men, osteoporosis".

Erectile dysfunctions in men are closely related to magnesium deficiency. Dr Sircus points out that transdermal supplementation of magnesium leads to a boost of magnesium in the body and an increase in DHEA and testosterone, which helps to improve the sexual function and libido, both in men and women.

Transdermal magnesium supplementation normalises levels of DHEA and boosts levels of testosterone in men and to a smaller extent in women. It balances the levels of estrogen and progesterone in women, thus reducing menopausal symptoms, menstrual problems, PMT, development of pre-eclampsia in pregnant women.

A boost in magnesium levels through transdermal supplementation is fast and free of side-effects which sometimes arise with oral supplementation. Because of the speed with which magnesium levels are replenished through transdermal procedures, the effects of it can be felt quickly on all levels, including reproductive function both in men and women.

Dr Sircus writes, referring to a study in Japan: "In men, decreased levels of magnesium gives rise to vasoconstriction from increased thromboxane level, increased endothelial intracellular calcium, and decreased nitric oxide. This may lead to premature emission and ejaculation processes. Magnesium is also probably involved in semen transport." (Magnesium for Life, 2007, p.244).

Dr Sircus's talks about the topical application of magnesium oil to reproductive organs regularly, especially just before having sex. Such applications would relax the tissues and quickly increase blood circulation in the area, both in men and women. It would also promote vaginal lubrication and relaxation of the muscles in the vagina, which would help eliminate the sensation of pain and discomfort during sex. In men, it would lead to a relaxation of the blood vessels supplying the penis, an increase in the blood flow and sensation in the area, and a stronger, longer-lasting erection.

Considering that the effect of such an application is so profound both in men and women, it is difficult to understand why this has not been publicised on a much wider scale. The market is flooded with legally and illegally-produced medicines loaded with dangerous side-effects, and magnesium is not only free from side-effects but is needed by the body in large quantities.

Transdermal applications increase absorption of magnesium into the body, dilate blood vessels, relax muscles and body tissues, increase peripheral circulation, improve tissue sensitivity and fluid secretions.

Unit 2 - Magnesium for Girls & Women - Adolescence and Pregnancy

Magnesium plays a very important role in a woman's body. Every stage of a woman's life is linked to the high requirements of magnesium. Childhood, adolescence, pregnancy, the menopause, and the age of maturity - all of these create their challenges and requirements.

Throughout a woman's reproductive life, the body undergoes constant hormonal changes. Ovulation, menstruation, pregnancy, childbirth, lactation, the menopause - all of these put a lot of strain on a woman's body.

Hormone production requires a lot of magnesium, and the woman's physiology means higher requirements in it. Magnesium deficiencies lead to hormonal imbalances, which in turn result in disturbances of body processes in a woman's body.

On the other hand, hormonal changes lead to changes in magnesium levels. Oestrogen and progesterone rise during ovulation and menstruation lead to higher demands on magnesium, which decreases its levels in the body.

A study of 19 women suffering from PMS has concluded that magnesium level decrease in women-sufferers as opposed to non-sufferers. (Biological Psychiatry Volume 35, Issue 8, 15 April 1994, Pages 557-561).

We have all heard of women craving chocolate just before the period is due. Dark chocolate is abundant with magnesium, and the body instinctively chooses the food containing it. It has been said to help with cramps and moodiness associated with PMS. Magnesium is a natural relaxant, so is irreplaceable in relaxing muscles and relieving menstrual cramps, which have been researched to be linked to magnesium deficiency.

Pregnancy puts an enormous strain on the woman's body, with extra requirements of minerals not only for the mother but also for the developing child. Magnesium deficiency in pregnancy may lead to a very dangerous condition called pre-eclampsia which may lead to eclampsia - both conditions are associated with hypertension (high blood pressure).

Magnesium Sulphate (Epsom Salt) has been used in the treatment of women with pre-eclampsia for many decades. In hospitals, it is administered intravenously. However, many pregnant women use it transdermally, by taking Epsom Salt baths regularly.

Transdermal application of magnesium means that the body regulates magnesium intake and will absorb the amount naturally required. Of course, it does not mean that a woman with any serious condition should resort to self-treatment. Magnesium baths are a preventative measure, and should not be used by women or natural health practitioners as a treatment.

Magnesium entering the woman's body invariably benefits the child. It has been suggested that prenatal magnesium administration may reduce the risk of cerebral palsy for very low birthweight babies. (Nelson K. Magnesium sulfate and risk of cerebral palsy in very-low-birth-weight infants. JAMA. 1996;276:1843–1844).

However, where magnesium is administered to a pregnant woman intravenously, it can also cause hypermagnesemia in babies with such symptoms as flaccidity, hyporeflexia, and respiratory depression. (Lipsitz PJ. The clinical and biochemical effects of excess magnesium in the newborn. Paediatrics. 1971;47:501–509).

A scientific study has shown that dietary magnesium deficiency in rats has resulted in a failure to lactate and

impaired growth and development in their offspring.
http://jn.nutrition.org/content/113/12/2421.full.pdf

This shows that magnesium is a crucial element required at various stages in a woman's life, especially the ones which are associated with her reproductive function.

Caution: Pregnant and lactating women should always seek medical advice before using oral or other forms of magnesium supplementation. There are also other contra-indications and cautions which although rare, should be considered by people at risk before any supplementation.

Unit 3 - Premenstrual Tension (PMT) and Magnesium

Several scientific studies have linked pre-menstrual tension - PMT (also called Pre-menstrual Syndrome) - with magnesium deficiency in a woman's body.

Premenstrual syndrome (PMS) shows itself as a group of physical and emotional symptoms which some women experience 1-2 weeks before their menstrual period. Normally, these symptoms subside when the period starts and within a couple of days of menstrual flow.

Statistics indicate that PMS affects over 80% of women of the reproductive age at some point in their lives, and about 40% of women experience symptoms bad enough to affect their daily life.

The symptoms may include, but are not limited to, stomach cramps, dizziness, tender breasts, water retention & swelling of the body, abdominal bloating, food cravings, especially for chocolate, nausea, vomiting, stomach upsets, appetite changes, insomnia, general discomfort, anger, irritability, crying seemingly for no reason, aches and pains all over the body, fatigue, lowered immunity, and many other symptoms.

Facchinetti F, Borella P, Sances G, Fioroni L, Nappi RE, Genazzani AR report the following results of a 2-months' study of 32 women-sufferers from PMS:

"To evaluate the effects of an oral Mg preparation on premenstrual symptoms, we studied, by a double-blind, randomized design, 32 women (24-39 years old) with PMS confirmed by the Moos Menstrual Distress Questionnaire. After 2 months of baseline recording, the subjects were randomly assigned to placebo or Mg for two cycles. In the next two cycles, both groups received Mg. Magnesium pyrrolidone carboxylic acid (360 mg Mg) or placebo was administered three times a day, from the 15th day of the menstrual cycle to the onset of menstrual flow.

Blood samples for Mg measurement were drawn premenstrually, during the baseline period, and in the second and fourth months of treatment. The Menstrual Distress Questionnaire score of the cluster "pain" was significantly reduced during the second month in both groups, whereas Mg treatment significantly affected both the total Menstrual Distress Questionnaire score and the cluster "negative effect."

In the second month, the women assigned to treatment showed a significant increase in Mg in lymphocytes and polymorphonuclear cells, whereas no changes were observed in plasma and erythrocytes. These data indicate that Mg supplementation could represent an effective treatment of premenstrual symptoms related to mood changes." http://www.ncbi.nlm.nih.gov/pubmed/2067759

"Three small double-blind RCTs have investigated the effect of magnesium supplementation in PMS. A trial in 38 women with relatively mild PMS found that a daily supplement of 200mg of magnesium reduced one out of six studied symptom categories. Fluid retention was significantly reduced in the second, but not the first month of use, but there were no significant effects on emotional symptoms...

Supplementation with magnesium 360mg/day in 32 women significantly reduced total PMS symptoms, specifically those related to mood,23 while in another trial in 20 women with

a premenstrual migraine, the same dose of magnesium significantly reduced the number of days with a headache."
http://www.pms.org.uk/About+PMS/News/
2007+bulletins/August+2007/item820/

The complexities of the reproductive cycle mean that the body mobilises itself for possible fertilization and pregnancy. This preparation leads to several hormones being produced in large quantities, and released into the body, leading to physiological and psychological changes in all the body systems. Magnesium plays a very important role not only in the production of hormones but as an integral part of ATP - the energy molecule of every cell.

Premenstrual activity in the woman's body requires a lot of magnesium. If it is in short supply, then certain processes are slowed down, and general physical and psychological tension, fatigue, cramps, aches, pain, lack of energy follow as just some of the numerous symptoms of what we call Premenstrual Tension.

Chocolate craving just before the period is nothing but a sign that the body needs magnesium. Eating dark chocolate alone will not solve the problem - magnesium needs to get into the body regularly in the form of nuts, seeds, green leafy vegetables and seafood (where possible). Magnesium also needs to come into the body in the form of supplements - in a vitamin form or transdermal application of magnesium salts.

Unit 4 - Stress, Fertility and Magnesium

Taking it easy may be the offhand advice doctors give to women who cannot conceive, but new scientific evidence confirms that stress does indeed play a role in conception.

Researchers at Oxford University and the US National Institutes of Health measured stress in women trying to get pregnant and found that those who were most stressed were least likely to conceive.

Stress joins other well-known pregnancy risk factors such as excessive alcohol consumption, smoking and obesity. The study measured two stress hormones in healthy women between the ages of 18 and 40 who were trying to conceive. It found that women with high levels of adrenaline had a 12 percent lower chance of conceiving when fertile as compared to those who were less stressed.

"Irrespective of the day or frequency of sexual intercourse during the fertile window, women with higher concentrations of alpha-amylase were less likely to conceive than women with lower concentrations," the study said, referring to the enzyme that is an indicator of adrenalin levels.

However, women who were found to have a higher level of cortisol, which is a measure of chronic stress, were no less likely to conceive than women with lower levels of the stress hormone. Dr Cecilia Pyper, of the National Perinatal Epidemiology Unit at the University of Oxford, said: "The findings support the idea that couples should aim to stay as relaxed as they can about trying for a baby.

"In some people's cases, it might be relevant to look at relaxation techniques, counselling and even approaches like yoga and meditation."The findings are published in the journal Fertility and Sterility.
http://uk.health.lifestyle.yahoo.net/stress-and-fertility.htm

Of course, yoga and relaxation, as well as other ways to slow down and relax the body and mind are immensely beneficial, but when I read this article, I thought to myself that without magnesium supplementation relaxation techniques will only have a limited effect.

Magnesium is possibly the most powerful natural relaxant which gets depleted when we are under stress. It takes part in numerous body processes - over 300 chemical reactions. It is essential in the production of the hormones related to fertility and normal sexual function.

Extreme or long-term chronic stress can lead to disturbances in the menstrual cycle, failing to ovulate, and infertility. The reason is that stress disturbs the production of fertility hormones. Stress affects both male and female reproductive function, so it is important to address the problem of infertility on both sides.

Just like with other hormones, production of fertility hormones depends on a sufficient amount of magnesium in the body. Magnesium is also required for the production of healthy sperm and egg. So, if you are trying to conceive, among other things, do make sure that your magnesium level is in balance - man or woman.

Module 14 - Magnesium Requirements for Different Groups of People

Unit 1 - Magnesium for Different Age Groups

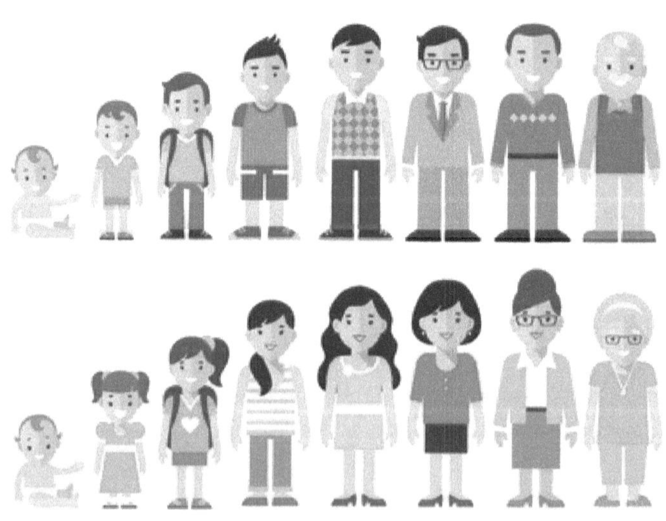

Magnesium deficiency is a common fact not just in adults, but increasingly in children of all ages, including very young kids. If a nursing mother is deficient in magnesium, the infant will most probably be deficient too. This will show itself as poor sleep, excitability, frequent crying, and sometimes even as more serious symptoms which should always be addressed by a doctor.

Academic pressures, athletic performance demands on a growing body, hormonal changes, peer pressure leading to stress - all of these factors mean that our children are using up lots of magnesium, and modern nutrient-poor diet with much of it being junk food, lack of exercise, over-consumption of sugar-loaded fizzy drinks and even alcohol make the problem much much worse.

Combined with the fact that the soil and water in most parts of the world are deficient in magnesium, we have increasing rates in depression, anxiety, ADHD (Attention Deficit Hyperactivity Disorder), general tension in the body, juvenile delinquency, poor response to stressful situations, low energy levels, cardiac disorders, hypertension, childhood obesity, poor immunity, behaviour and many other conditions.

Multiple challenges which our children have to face at home, school and in the streets mean that a lot of magnesium is being used by the body with the production of adrenaline and other hormones. This has resulted in an increase in mental disorders, such as depression and ADHD (Attention Deficit Hyperactivity Disorder).

Alcohol consumption by children is also on the increase. Alcohol is the biggest "thief" of magnesium damaging the liver, heart, kidneys and brain. Alcohol-dependent children are much more likely to suffer liver damage, heart disease, depression and premature death. Alcohol is especially damaging for girls, leading to an increase in breast cancer rate later in life.

Childhood depression is another growing problem linked to magnesium deficiency. Serotonin - the hormone of happiness - is reliant on sufficient stocks of magnesium in the body. Anti-depressants prescribed to children deplete magnesium levels even further.

As we mature, our requirement in magnesium increases, and in many people - deficiency too. This happens due to lifestyle issues (insufficient sleep, alcohol abuse, smoking, too much junk food and drink), mineral-poor soil in the area, drinking soft water, increased physical and psychological demands, inability to respond effectively to challenging situations and poor adaptation to change, poor environment, a general state of health, reliance on medication - all of these factors can deplete magnesium very quickly.

As we grow even older, a lack of this important mineral becomes a real issue and is reflected in premature ageing, excess weight, brittle bones, wrinkles, lack of energy, poor sleep and other factors that prevent us from enjoying our lives to a good old age.

Magnesium is such an important mineral that even minor deficiency shows itself in various ways quite soon, so supplementing it regularly is essential to the health of people of all ages.

Unit 2 - Sport and Magnesium

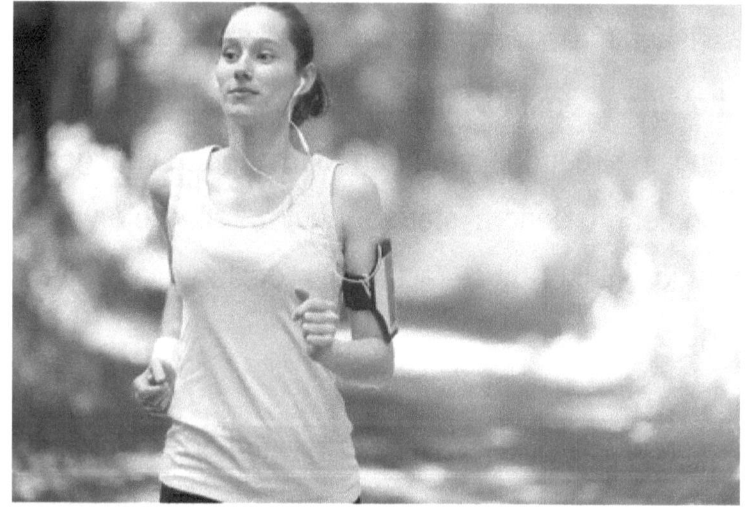

As I've mentioned earlier, magnesium plays a vital role in our lives. It is an irreplaceable component in the production of energy from ATP - the molecule which provides energy for all body processes and movements. If magnesium is depleted there is not enough of it for energy production which means that metabolic processes do not get sufficient energy, so general metabolism slows down resulting in energy slumps. **An increase in magnesium levels in the body increases general energy and performance.**

Another important function of magnesium is connected with its interaction with calcium in the body. Calcium ensures muscle contraction, and an excessive amount of calcium leads to muscle spasms, cramps, muscle tension, as well as tightness in the joints. If calcium ensures contraction and strength of the muscle then the role of magnesium is to relax all body tissues, including muscles, nerves, the brain, heart, blood vessels, etc.

Needless to say, **insufficient magnesium results in all-round rigidity and stress**. If there is too much calcium circulating in the body it binds with fat in the blood with the potential to form atheromas leading to the narrowing of blood vessels, increase in the blood pressure and danger of them breaking away and blocking the arteries. Lack of sufficient magnesium reduces the elasticity of the blood vessels resulting in arteriosclerosis, which is also a contributing factor towards high blood pressure.

Athletes are especially prone to magnesium losses and resulting deficiency which can lead to reduced performance, muscle rigidity, tetany, cramps, decreased endurance, general weakness, as well as an array of cardiovascular problems such as an increase in blood pressure, arrhythmia and rigidity of the blood vessels.

While short high-intensity exercise leads to an increase of magnesium levels (hypermagnesemia), due to a shift of magnesium from the cells into the plasma as a result of acidosis and a general decrease of plasma levels, prolonged exercise leads to depletion of plasma magnesium (hypomagnesemia).

A few reasons for magnesium losses during prolonged sports activities have been suggested:

1. Lipolysis (fat metabolism). Fatty acids are mobilised for energy production during exercise which leads to magnesium deficiency.
2. General physical and psychological stress on all body systems during prolonged exercise.
3. Loss of magnesium through sweating - this normally happens in humid hot conditions.
4. Loss of magnesium in urine during intensive short-term exercise activities.

Magnesium losses are especially substantial during periods of **training for sporting events**.

"Several studies indicate that there is a sustained fall in plasma Mg concentration after strenuous exercise and that hypomagnesaemia either persists or worsens during a season of training 21,46,47,48, a sound reason for looking more carefully at the Mg intake of athletes. A recent longitudinal study of a group of medium-distance runners carried out over a training season also demonstrated plasma Mg reductions during the competition period, although there were no variations in erythrocyte Mg. Since both their energy intake and their workload remained more or less constant during the study, a relationship can be established between plasma Mg changes and the stress of the competition period 4" (Y. Rayssiguier1, C. Y. Guezennec2, and J. Durlach3, New experimental and clinical data on the relationship between magnesium and sport, http://www.mgwater.com/dur18.shtml)

Another study has established a **link between stress, magnesium deficiency and the immune response:** "Physical exercise may deplete Mg, which together with a marginal dietary Mg intake may impair immune function [4]. Strenuous exercise induces immunodepression that is multifactorial in origin. Aspects of immune function can be depressed temporarily by either a single bout of very severe exercise or a longer period of excessive training. Depressed immunity may allow an episode of infection, particularly upper respiratory tract infections. Thus, the ability to perform physical work may be compromised.

Strenuous exercise induces petrogenesis and suppresses cellular immunity leading to increased susceptibility to infections [22]. A common view is that Upper Respiratory Tract Infections (URTI) are increased in elite endurance athletes after single bouts of endurance exercise and during intensive training. The evidence is inconclusive, although exercise does alter the number and function of circulating innate immune cells [23]. Lymphocytosis is observed during and immediately after exercise, proportional to exercise intensity and duration, before returning to resting values normally within 24 h. Mobilization of T and B cell subsets is largely influenced by catecholamines. This apparent depression in acquired immunity appears to be related to exercise-induced elevated stress hormones. Salivary IgA underlying the alterations in mucosal immunity with acute exercise is probably under the control of the sympathetic nervous system. There are numerous examples where exercise alters measures of immunity by 15-25% [23].

As with Mg studies, inflammatory markers escalate with strenuous exercise. CRP and TNFα increased significantly during the two weeks of exercise [24]. Four days of increased training load reduced running performance and altered the inflammatory response to high-intensity intermittent exercise [25]. CRP is higher is contact sport than noncontact [26] and in exercising females compared to males [27].

Differences in the immune responses to exercise between healthy and illness-prone athletes may explain the greater incidence of URTI. The relationship between resting CRP concentrations and the peak pro and anti-inflammatory responses to exercise support involvement of CRP in the complex network regulating exercise-induced inflammatory disturbances [28]. Excessive cytokine release related to overtraining [29] may upset the balance between modulation of repair and development of inflammation and possible infections."
http://www.omicsonline.org/magnesium-influence-on-stress-and-immune-function-in-exercise-2161-0673.1000111.pdf

Magnesium deficiency may play a role in **sudden death syndrome** in sportspeople resulting from a cardiac arrest (heart attack). As we have established earlier, a fall in magnesium levels in sportspeople can lead to an increase in cholesterol, blood sugar levels, and rigidity of blood vessels due to a calcium-magnesium imbalance which in turn results in an increase in blood pressure and may in some cases explain sudden death in athletes.

All this brings us to a conclusion that it is extremely important to replenish magnesium levels in athletes, especially during prolonged sporting activities and competitions, to prevent a slump in energy levels, general fatigue, reduction in performance, muscle tension, aches and pains and speed up recovery.

Module 15 - Vitamins and Minerals that Work in Synergy with Magnesium

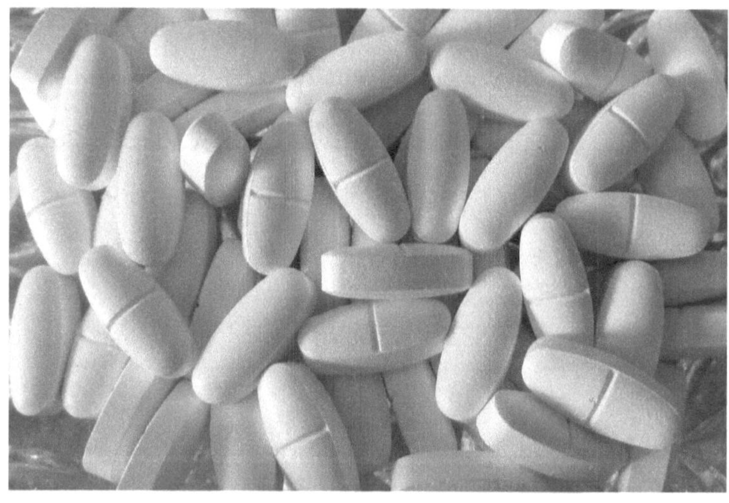

Unit 1 - Calcium-Magnesium Synergy

For decades now, a message has been pushed by doctors and health organisations urging people, especially children, to drink more milk and eat products containing calcium - to ensure healthy teeth and prevent osteoporosis in later stages in life.

Products such as cereals are being fortified with calcium. However, despite a record-high consumption of milk in the developed world, more and more people are diagnosed as suffering from osteoporosis and as having poor dental health. Why is it so?

The fact is, we have not been told one very important fact in all this time - that calcium works in synergy with magnesium. They are antagonists, and one cannot work without the other. If we consume just calcium without balancing it with magnesium, our cells, blood vessels and organs will eventually become hard like stone, due to deposition of calcium in them. But of course, it can only happen in theory, since in practice this imbalance will quickly lead to the blood vessels and body organs failing. In practice, calcium-magnesium imbalance leads to muscle spasms, deposition of plaque in arteries which leads to high blood pressure, cardiac problems and even death.

In her book "The Miracle of Magnesium" Dr Carolyn Dean writes: "I've heard statistics like a 700 percent rise in osteoporosis in 10 years, even while taking all this calcium. The myth that's been created about calcium is that we need twice as much calcium as we do magnesium. Most of the supplements reflect this. We've got a situation where people are taking 1,200 to 1,500 milligrams of calcium and maybe a few hundred milligrams of magnesium." The ratio of calcium to magnesium needs to be 1:1 rather than 2:1, Dr Dean says.

In the same chapter, she continues: "Research shows that the ratio of calcium to magnesium in the palaeolithic diet - the ancient diet that had evolved with our bodies - was 1:1, compared with 5:1 to 15:1 ratio in the present diets. With an average of ten times more calcium than magnesium in our current diet, there is no doubt about widespread magnesium deficiency in modern times... In our society we tend to look for "the best", "the most important", "the star" and forget that it takes a team and teamwork to get anything accomplished, including body processes. Calcium, because it is the most abundant mineral in the body, therefore became "the star". Even though research has accumulated on magnesium over the past four decades, it has never been adequately publicised or discussed".

Unit 2 - Vitamins D and K2

While it is necessary to observe the magnesium-calcium ratio, we also need to remember that these minerals work in synergy with vitamins K and D2. This is what Dr Mercola writes on the subject:

"I want to remind you that calcium and magnesium also need to be balanced with vitamin D and K2. Many of Dr Dean's blogs address this issue and her concern that high dose vitamin D can overwork magnesium and lead to magnesium deficiency.

These four nutrients [magnesium, calcium, vitamins D and K2 - PNC] perform an intricate dance together, with one supporting the other. Lack of balance between these nutrients is why calcium supplements have become associated with increased risk of heart attacks and stroke, and why some people experience vitamin D toxicity.

Part of the explanation for these adverse side effects is that vitamin K2 keeps calcium in its appropriate place. If you're K2 deficient, added calcium can cause more problems than it solves, by accumulating in the wrong places.

Similarly, if you opt for oral vitamin D, you need to also consume it in your food or take supplemental vitamin K2 and more magnesium. Taking mega doses of vitamin D supplements without sufficient amounts of K2 and magnesium can lead to vitamin D toxicity and magnesium deficiency symptoms, which include inappropriate calcification.

Magnesium and vitamin K2 complement each other, as magnesium helps lower blood pressure, which is an important component of heart disease. So, all in all, anytime you're taking any of the following: magnesium, calcium, vitamin D3, or vitamin K2, you need to consider all the others as well, since these all work synergistically with one another".

http://articles.mercola.com/sites/articles/archive/2013/12/0
8/magnesium-health-benefits.aspx

Module 16 - Products Used In Transdermal Magnesium Therapy

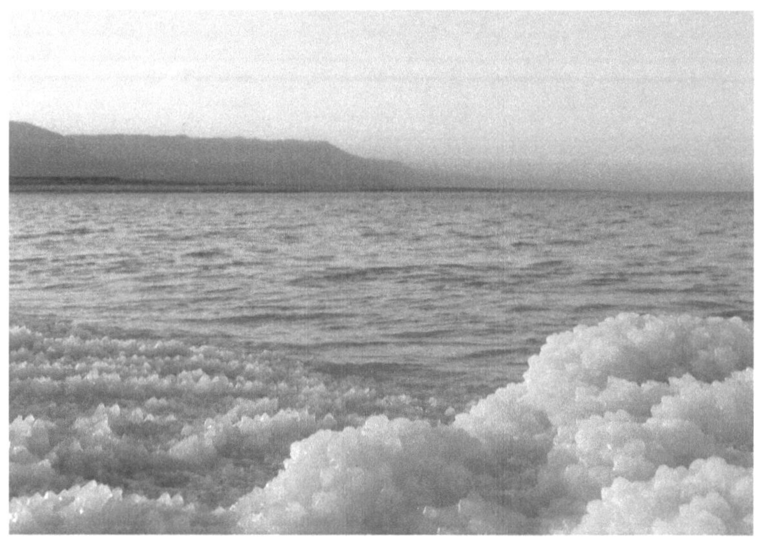

Unit 1 - Magnesium Chloride

Magnesium chloride comes in 2 forms - as crystalline flakes and as a highly concentrated solution, widely known as magnesium oil. Magnesium flakes are also known as magnesium chloride hexahydrate, with 6 molecules of water bound to 1 molecule of magnesium chloride: $MgCl_2(H_2O)_6$. This explains why the flakes "melt" in warm temperatures turning into an oil-like substance which is a highly concentrated salt solution.

Magnesium oil as we know it is also a highly concentrated magnesium chloride solution, but less so that the melted flakes would be. This is achieved by adding water to the salt, so the solution is still oily to the touch, but less so than the melted flakes.

Which product to use for which treatment?

Magnesium oil can be used for:

1. Magnesium oil massage
2. Magnesium body spray
3. Magnesium body wrap
4. Magnesium compress
5. Mouthwash (diluted with water)

6. Deodorant

7. Magnesium bath & foot bath (expensive, since a lot is needed)

8. Purified magnesium oil can be taken internally (care should be taken by people with certain health problems).

Magnesium flakes can be used for:

1. Magnesium bath and foot bath

2. To make magnesium oil with

3. Magnesium body wrap

4. Magnesium compress

5. Other applications used with magnesium oil.

This is a list of main applications for magnesium oil and flakes. However, it can be expanded depending on a person's needs. Make sure to check for contra-indications before any application.

Unit 2 - Making Magnesium Oil from Flakes

Magnesium oil made from flakes is of a lower quality than manufacturer-produced products. However, there are cases when magnesium oil may be unavailable or unaffordable, so in this unit, we will learn how to make magnesium oil from magnesium flakes.

The flakes are 47% magnesium chloride and about 50.5% water. A 33% solution means that there will be 33% magnesium chloride. So, **100 grams of flakes (which contain 50.5 grams of water) will need an extra 42 grams of water**. (1g of water equals 1ml of water).The 47 grams of magnesium chloride will then be dissolved in 142 grams of solution, giving the 33% strength that is required.

This can be scaled up to a convenient batch size - every kilogram of flakes will require 420 grams of water to be added to it to get a 33% strength used in commercially available magnesium oil. It will take some time to dissolve magnesium oil in water, so the quickest thing to do is to mix it with hot water and leave it to dissolve.

An easier way to make magnesium oil is to mix 1 part of flakes with 1 part of warm water (for example, 100g of flakes with 100ml of water). It will produce a less concentrated solution which will suit sensitive and dry skin type.

Unit 3 - Magnesium Sulphate (Epsom Salt)

Magnesium sulphate heptahydrate $MgSO_4 \cdot 7H_2O$ - otherwise known as Epsom salt - is a great alternative to magnesium chloride. It is well-known for its pain and tension-relieving properties. The basis of the product is formed by a magnesium sulphate molecule bound by 7 molecules of water. So like magnesium chloride, is it a "watery" salt which can melt in hot temperatures.

Anhydrous magnesium sulfate is used as a drying agent. Since the anhydrous form is hygroscopic (readily absorbs water from the air) and therefore harder to weigh accurately, the hydrate is often preferred when preparing solutions, for example in medical preparations. Epsom salts have traditionally been used as a component of bath salts.

What is the difference between magnesium chloride and magnesium sulphate?

I have been asked many times about the **differences between magnesium chloride and magnesium sulphate**, *commonly known as* **Epsom Salts**. *There is a great article about it written by Dr Mark Sircus, a well-known and recognised researcher of magnesium and its benefits. I quote it here:*

"According to Daniel Reid, author of The Tao of Detox, magnesium sulfate, commonly known as Epsom salts, is rapidly excreted through the kidneys and therefore difficult to assimilate. This would explain in part why the effects of Epsom salt baths do not last long and why you need more magnesium sulfate in a bath than magnesium chloride to get similar results.

Magnesium chloride is easily assimilated and metabolized in the human body.[1] However, Epsom salts are used specifically by parents of children with autism because of the sulfate, which they are usually deficient in, sulfate is also crucial to the body and is wasted in the urine of autistic children.

For cellular detoxification and tissue purification, the most effective form of magnesium is magnesium chloride, which has a strong excretory effect on toxins and stagnant energies stuck in the tissues of the body, drawing them out through the pores of the skin.

This is a powerful hydrotherapy that draws toxins from the tissues, replenishes the "vital fluid" of the cells and restores cellular magnesium to optimum levels. Magnesium Chloride is environmentally safe and is used around vegetation and in agriculture. It is not irritating to the skin at lower concentrations and is less toxic than common table salt.

Magnesium Chloride solution was not only harmless for tissues, but it had also a great effect on leucocytic activity and phagocytosis; so it was perfect for external wounds treatment.

Dr Jean Durlach et al, at the Université P. et M. Curie, Paris, wrote a paper about the relative toxicities between magnesium sulfate and magnesium chloride. They write, "The reason of the toxicity of magnesium pharmacological doses of magnesium using the sulfate anion rather than the chloride anion may perhaps arise from the respective chemical structures of both the two magnesium salts. Chemically, both $MgSO_4$ and $MgCl_2$ are hexa-aqueous complexes.

However $MgCl_2$ crystals consist of dianions with magnesium coordinated to the six water molecules as a complex, $[Mg(H_2O)_6]^{2+}$ and two independent chloride anions, Cl^-. In $MgSO_4$, a seventh water molecule is associated with the sulphate anion, $[Mg(H_2O)_6]^{2+}[SO_4 \cdot H_2O]$. Consequently, the more hydrated $MgSO_4$ molecule may have chemical interactions with paracellular components, rather than with cellular components, presumably potentiating toxic manifestations while reducing the therapeutic effect."

$MgSO_4$ is not always the appropriate salt in clinical therapeutics. $MgCl_2$ seems the better anion-cation association to be used in many clinical and pharmacological indications.[2] Dr Jean Durlach et al.

Magnesium sulfate is a chemical compound containing magnesium and sulfate, with the formula $MgSO_4$. In its hydrated form, the pH is 6.0 (5.5 to 7.0). It is often encountered as the heptahydrate, $MgSO_4 \cdot 7H_2O$, commonly called Epsom salts. Anhydrous magnesium sulfate is used as a drying agent. Since the anhydrous form is hygroscopic (readily absorbs water from the air) and therefore harder to weigh accurately, the hydrate is often preferred when preparing solutions, for example in medical preparations. Epsom salts have traditionally been used as a component of bath salts.

Therapeutic & home uses of Epsom salt

- Bath
- Footbath
- Body wrap
- Magnesium compress
- Mouthwash (diluted with water)
- Purified magnesium sulphate can be taken internally for detox purposes - under medical observation.

References:

[1] http://www.hps-online.com/foodprof14.htm

[2] Magnesium Research. Volume 18, Number 3, 187-92, September 2005, original article"

http://magnesiumforlife.com/product-information/magnesium-chloride-vs-magnesium-sulfate/

Unit 4 - Dead Sea Salt

The Dead Sea as it is today was formed over billions of

years, as a result of continuous evaporation of seawater, which has happened because the sea has no connection with the ocean at present. The Dead Sea is one of the most ancient seas on Earth, based 400 metres below the sea level.

The process of evaporation of the water from the Dead Sea has produced a phenomenon which lives up to its name since no life can survive in the highly saline environment of Dead Sea.

The Dead Sea is incredibly rich in minerals. It contains all the essential elements of the Periodic table which are encountered and used by the body and countless other healing substances. **Magnesium chloride** forms a large percentage of mineral salts in it. The Dead Sea is, in fact, the most common source of magnesium chloride on the market.

Extensive scientific research has demonstrated excellent results for its effectiveness in the treatment of various skin problems such as acne, psoriasis, dermatitis, eczema.

Because of its high levels of magnesium and bromide, the salt has been used widely to treat nervous disorders and musculoskeletal complaints, such as arthritis, as well as inflammatory conditions of all body systems.

Dead Sea salt is used to treat the following:

- Eczema, psoriasis, dermatitis
- Acne, spots, oily skin - balancing
- Ageing, sagging, sallow skin - rejuvenation
- Inflammatory conditions
- Rheumatoid arthritis
- Muscle aches, pains
- Back pain
- Poor circulation
- Bruising
- Sprains, strains
- General fatigue & debility
- Stress-related conditions
- Ulcers
- Nervous disorders
- Respiratory problems

- Obesity.

Suggested applications

- Body wraps (same as above)
- Baths (use 500g per bath)
- Compresses (mix 1 part of salt with 3 parts of water, soak a cloth, apply on the area, wrap with clingfilm and a warm scarf. Leave on for 2 hours or overnight.)
- Footbaths (use 100-150g per footbath per 6-7 litres of warm water to relieve aching feet, improve circulation and help with leg ulcers).

Module 17 - Transdermal Therapy - How Does It Work? The Skin - Structure & Functions.

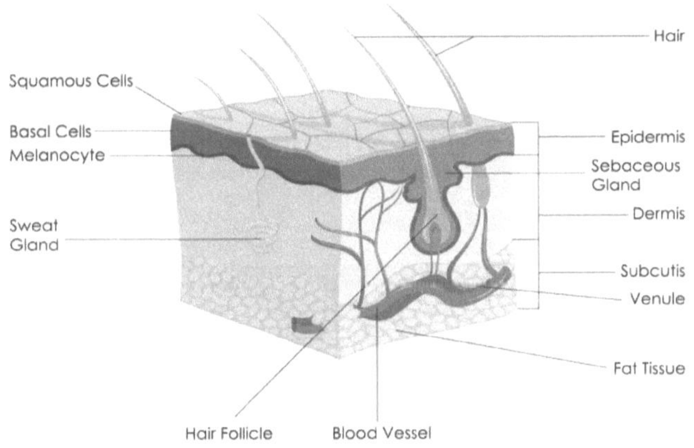

Unit 1 - The Skin - Structure & Functions

The skin is a remarkable organ of the body which can perform various vital functions. It can mould to different shapes, stretch and harden, but can also feel a delicate touch, pain, pressure, hot and cold, and is an effective communicator between the outside environment and the brain.

The skin makes up to 12-15% of an adult's body weight. Each square centimetre has 6 million cells, 5,000 sensory points, 100 sweat glands and 15 sebaceous glands. It consists of 3 layers: the epidermis (the outer layer), the dermis ('true skin') and the subcutaneous (fat) layer.

The skin is constantly being regenerated. A skin cell starts its life at the lower layer of the skin (the basal layer of the dermis), which is supplied with blood vessels and nerve ending. The cell migrates upward for about two weeks until it reaches the bottom portion of the epidermis, which is the outermost skin layer.

The epidermis is not supplied with blood vessels but has nerve endings. For another 2 weeks, the cell undergoes a series of changes in the epidermis, gradually flattening out and moving toward the surface. Then it dies and is shed. Below is a detailed diagram of the skin structure:

Epidermis

The main function of the epidermis is to form a tough barrier against between the body and the outside world, while the dermis is a soft, thick cushion of connective tissue that lies directly below the epidermis and largely determines the way our skin looks.

Both layers keep repairing and renewing themselves throughout or life, but the dermis does it more slowly than the epidermis. Under the dermis is a layer of fat cells, which is known as adipose tissue (or subcutaneous fat layer). It provides insulation and protective padding for the body. It also provides an emergency energy supply.

The epidermis consists of 5 layers:

1. The basal layer (Stratum germinativum) - this is the bottom layer of the skin. The cells of this layer constantly been reproduced, since they contain a nucleus or seed. As the cells reproduce, the layers get constantly pushed up into the next layer.

2. The prickle cell layer (Stratum spinosum) - called this way because the cells have spines which prevent bacteria from entering the cells and moisture being lost. These cells also have a nucleus and therefore reproduce.

3. The granular layer (Stratum granulosum) - the prickle cells lose their spines and become flattened. The nucleus dies, and protein is formed called keratin. This protein prevents moisture loss and is found in skin, nails and hair.

4. The clear layer (Stratum lucidum) - this layer is for cushioning and protection and is found only on the palms of the hands and soles of the feet.

5. The horny (cornified) layer (Stratum corneum) - the cells here are dead and ready to be shed (desquamation). This process speeds up as we age.

Dermis

The dermis is the layer responsible for the skin's structural integrity, elasticity and resilience. Wrinkles develop in the dermis. Therefore, an anti-wrinkle treatment has a chance to succeed only if it can reach the dermis.

Typical collagen and elastin creams, for example, never reach the dermis because collagen and elastin molecules are too large to penetrate the epidermis. Hence, contrary to what some manufacturers of such creams might claim, these creams have little effect on skin wrinkles.

The dermis is the middle layer of the skin located between the epidermis and subcutaneous tissue. It is the thickest of the skin layers and comprises a tight, sturdy mesh of collagen and elastin fibres. Both collagen and elastin are critically important skin proteins: collagen is responsible for the structural support and elastin for the resilience of the skin.

The key type of cells in the dermis is fibroblasts, which synthesize collagen, elastin and other structural molecules. The proper function of fibroblasts is highly important for overall skin health. The dermis also contains capillaries (tiny blood vessels) and lymph nodes which produce immune cells.

Blood capillaries are responsible for bringing oxygen and nutrients to the skin and removing carbon dioxide and products of cell metabolism (what we call waste matter). Lymph nodes are engaged in protecting the skin from invading microorganisms.

Finally, the dermis contains sebaceous glands, sweat glands, hair follicles and a small number of nerve and muscle cells. Sebaceous glands, based around hair follicles, produce sebum, an oily protective substance that lubricates the skin and hair and provides protection by forming an acid mantle when mixed with sweat. When the sebaceous gland produces too little sebum, as is common in older people, the skin becomes excessively dry and more prone to wrinkling. Too much of sebum, as is common in teenagers, often leads to acne.

The dermis is thicker than the epidermis but has fewer cells. It consists mainly of connective tissue which is made up of fibres of the proteins collagen and elastin and a non-fibrous gelatin-like material called ground substance or extracellular matrix.

Subcutaneous tissue

Subcutaneous tissue is the deepest layer of the skin located under the dermis and consisting mainly of fat cells. It acts as a shock absorber and heat insulator, protecting underlying tissues from cold and trauma.

The loss of subcutaneous tissue in later years leads to facial sag and makes wrinkles more visible. To counteract it, a cosmetic procedure where fat is taken from elsewhere in the body and injected into facial areas is common these days.

Skin Functions

There are 6 skin functions:

1. Sensation - the nerve endings in the skin identify touch, heat, cold, pain and light pressure.

2. Heat regulation - the skin helps to regulate the body temperature by sweating to cool the body down when it overheats and shivering creating 'goosebumps' when it is cold. Shivering closes the pores. The tiny hair that stands on end traps warm air and thus helps keep the body warm.

3. Absorption - absorption of ultraviolet rays from the sun helps to form vitamin D in the body, which is vital for bone formation. Some creams, essential oils and medicines (e.g. HRT, anti-smoking patches) can also be absorbed through the skin into the bloodstream.

4. Protection - the skin protects the body from ultraviolet light - too much of it is harmful to the body - by producing a pigment called melanin. It also protects us from the invasion of bacteria and germs by forming an acid mantle (formed by the skin sebum and sweat). This barrier also prevents moisture loss.

5. Excretion - waste products and toxins are eliminated from the body through the sweat glands. It is a very important function which helps to keep the body 'clean' from the inside.

6. Secretion - sebum and sweat are secreted onto the skin surface. The sebum keeps the skin lubricated and soft, and the sweat combines with the sebum to form an acid mantle which creates the right pH balance for the skin to fight off infection.

I would add another very important but frequently overlooked function to this list: **diagnostic**. The skin shows the state of our health. So, when we are ill or otherwise unhealthy, the skin will reflect it immediately. The toxic, congested, tired, stressed body will often have pale, unhealthy complexion. Deprived of proper nourishment and good oxygen supply due to inefficient circulation and elimination, it will be more prone to various skin problems.

Unit 2 - Transdermal Therapy - How Does It Work?

Transdermal therapies rely on 2 main functions of the skin to work:

1. Absorption
2. Excretion

Both functions are possible due to the permeability of the skin thanks to its microporous structure. A large number of pores allows the skin to absorb various salts. aroma oils and even larger organic molecules of medicines. This function is very important in terms of transdermal mineral supplementation.

The same pores also allow the skin to release toxins. Excretion is a process opposite to absorption, with the skin releasing unwanted substances and water out of the body. Without this ability, the body systems would fail very quickly, because the body systems will not be able to take the pressure.

The skin takes upon itself a very important function to rid the body of toxins bypassing other channels, such as the liver and kidneys. This is why in cases of severe skin damage (due to burns for example), the body systems can fail very quickly - especially the kidneys.

The skin is very large if laid out and stretched, which allows it to work very efficiently. Of course, the skin by itself would be nothing without the network of multiple capillaries take away toxins to the skin surface for elimination. The same network delivers important nutrients from the surface of the skin to the cells inside the body. Salt ions are easiest for the skin to absorb and excrete, due to their minute size.

They come out with sweat and get inside the body when it is sprayed, massaged or submerged in a salty solution.

And here we should mention another remarkable property of the skin - called "osmosis". No matter how salty the water is (e.g. Dead Sea water is over-saturated with salt), the skin will not take more salt than necessary (unlike when salt is taken orally).

The skin regulates the intake of salts in a very intelligent way, stopping any salt overload. This means that saltwater balance is maintained at all times if one relies on supplementing minerals transdermally, as opposed to oral supplementation. No matter how salty the water in the sea, we do not become "overdosed" with salt from swimming in it.

Thanks to these properties of the skin, transdermal therapy is a very safe way to top the body up with the minerals it requires, and releasing toxins, bypassing the kidneys, thus reducing the risk of damage to body organs.

Here is what Dr Mark Sircus says about transdermal methods of application: "Drugs enter different layers of skin via intramuscular, subcutaneous, or transdermal delivery methods. The most common ways to administer drugs are oral (swallowing an aspirin tablet), intramuscular (getting a flu shot in an arm muscle), subcutaneous (injecting insulin just under the skin), intravenous (receiving medicines through a vein), or transdermal (wearing a skin patch). It is not a surprise, when you consider the large surface area of the skin, that when you apply a substance to the entire body, rapid absorption and resultant effect is sufficient to put the transdermal administration on par with or even ahead of other methods of administering drugs. "

He then continues: "Medicines taken by mouth (oral) pass through the liver before they are absorbed into the bloodstream. Transdermal application bypasses the liver, entering the tissues and blood more directly. "
http://drsircus.com/medicine/magnesium/use-magnesium-oil

Further Reading

1. 6 Ways to Detox through Your Skin.
http://www.mindbodygreen.com/0-1683/6-Ways-to-Detox-Through-Your-Skin.html
2. Arsenic, Cadmium, Lead, and Mercury in Sweat: A Systematic Review. Margaret E. Sears et al.
http://www.hindawi.com/journals/jeph/2012/184745/
3. Mineral Supplements May Be Used Via the Skin.
http://www.naturalnews.com/010061_minerals_skin_supplements.html

Module 18 - Application Methods of Transdermal Magnesium Therapy (Part 1)

Unit 1 – Magnesium Oil Massage

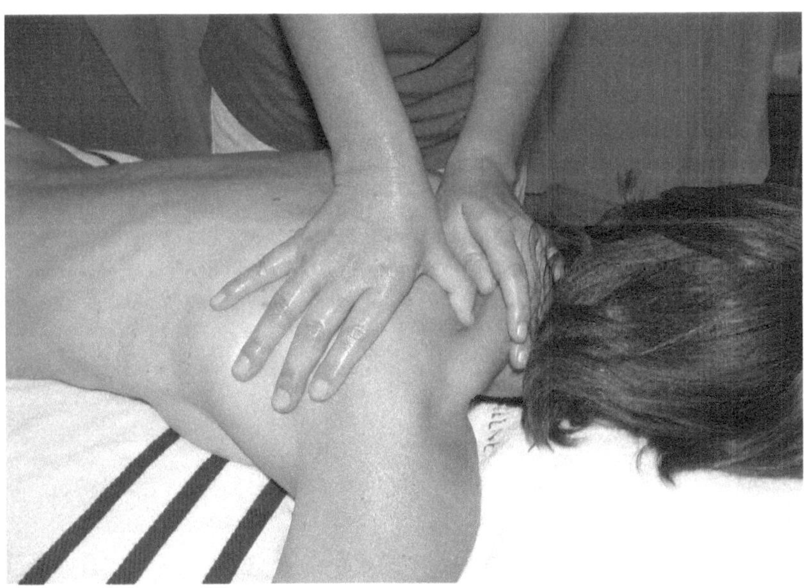

Magnesium oil has a light 'oily' texture, so can be easily

spread on the skin. This allows it to be used as a massage product. Magnesium oil massage is one of the most relaxing, deeply healing treatments anybody can receive. It works on both physical and psychological levels.

On the physical level it achieves the following results:

- Pain relief
- Reduction in cramps
- Improved mobility in the joints
- Improved circulation
- More energy
- Profound relaxation of all tissues
- Better sleep
- Improved metabolism
- Reduction in headaches
- More efficient elimination of toxic waste
- General improvement of health.

Massage can be done locally - on a specific area, or the whole body. Following are important things to take into account regarding magnesium massage:

- The best way to to do it is to warm up the product and the parts of the body being massaged. This can be done by using an infrared device or a hot water bottle for small areas.
- For larger areas or whole-body massage, a very warm shower can be taken before treatment. This will also hydrate the skin, which promotes the absorption of magnesium oil by it. A natural moisturiser can be used instead of a shower.
- Keeping the room and the body warm will promote relaxation and absorption of magnesium into the skin.
- For people with sensitive skin use sweet almond or another nut/seed oil before using magnesium oil.
- Adjust the length of treatment to your client's requirements.
- Magnesium massage can be done in a clinic or at home. One does not need special skills to do it for oneself or family members.
- Use gentle but firm strokes to rub the product into the skin focusing on areas of pain and discomfort.

- If you are a therapist, use the timing, techniques and procedures you use for therapeutic massage adjusting the treatment to your client's needs.

Remember that magnesium oil has a greater 'slip' than most nut/seed oils, so it may be difficult to use deep tissue techniques. So if your client requires those, you may want to start your treatment by using a nut/seed oil to work on areas of tension and rub magnesium oil on top of it later. But of course, it depends on your client's needs, and using just magnesium oil with lighter strokes may be just what is needed.

How often can a person have magnesium massage? Just like any other procedure with magnesium, massage can be used as often as needed, even daily. If a person shows signs of severe deficiency than it would be good to start with a daily massage which can later be scaled down to once every other day, twice a week and eventually once a week.

Unit 2 - Magnesium Bath

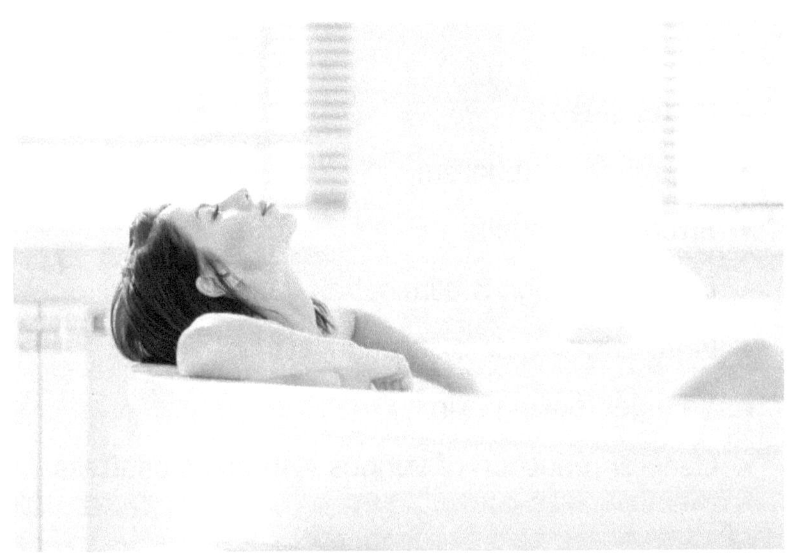

One of the most pleasant ways to replenish magnesium level is to take regular magnesium baths. Magnesium salt plus warm water work wonders for the body and mind. Such baths are thoroughly relaxing, bringing relief to an aching body and re-balancing all the body systems.

Therapeutic benefits of such baths are profound and accumulate as time goes by. These are just some of them:

- Mental relaxation
- Relaxation of the muscles
- Pain relief
- Better sleep
- Improved metabolism
- Stronger immunity
- Better digestion & elimination
- More effective detoxification
- Younger looking skin
- General reduction of various symptoms of stress.

One needs to remember though that it is not the fastest way to bring magnesium into the body unless a lot of magnesium salt is added to the water. For this purpose a magnesium massage, body spray or wrap would be more effective. However, magnesium baths have many benefits which other applications cannot offer, so by all means - do include them in your routine.

Here is what you would need:

- A bathful of warm water
- 250-350g of magnesium salt (more salt - 1kg or over - will enhance the effects).
- A towel.

For magnesium salt, use either magnesium flakes or Epsom salt (cheaper than flakes). Both are very effective, and Epsom salt has an added benefit – it binds toxins in the body, although magnesium from the flakes is more readily available to the body since the molecule is much lighter and the salt provides more magnesium for the same weight.

How long and how often?

How long you stay in the bath depends on how you feel about it. I'd say 20-30 minutes, but if you are very tired and achy, 40 minutes might bring better results (with an occasional addition of warm water). These baths can be taken daily if desired or at least twice a week for a long-term effect.

Unit 3 - Magnesium Foot Bath

Footbaths with magnesium salts are a quick, convenient and economical way to deliver magnesium to the body. The effect is not as profound as from the use of a full-body bath, magnesium wrap or an application of magnesium oil over the body. However, they are still effective in achieving the following goals:

1. Profound relaxation of the body tissues
2. Mental relaxation
3. Relief from pain and muscle tension (mostly in the feet and lower legs)
4. Relief from cramps
5. Improved circulation
6. Transdermal magnesium supplementation
7. Better sleep.

To make a foot bath, we will need 6-7 litres of warm water of about 46-47 degrees C. Warmer temperatures may be more effective, but it is important to remember that everyone has his or her temperature tolerance level, so it needs to be adjusted to an individual. We will also need about 150-200g of magnesium salt. More can be added if desired - it will enhance the effects. Add the salt to the water, mix it and put feet in the solution, for 20-30 minutes. Warm water can be added throughout the footbath if necessary.

Magnesium chloride, magnesium sulphate or the Dead Sea salt can be used for a footbath. It is important to remember that not every person can take a full-body bath, for whatever reason. A magnesium footbath offers a great alternative to achieving results similar to a bath, only on a smaller scale. And it can be enjoyed as often as you want.

Unit 4 - Magnesium Compress

A magnesium compress is a very effective way of soothing aches and pain. Following an injury, it is important to seek medical help immediately to exclude damage to the brain, bones, ligaments, other internal tissues and organs. A cold compress, such as an ice pack, is normally applied to an acute injury before help arrives. If it is a minor injury, then an ice pack may be sufficient.

For pain caused by a sudden injury, a magnesium compress is unsuitable in the first 2 days, since magnesium dilates blood vessels and may cause a haematoma (blood escaping into the surrounding tissues). It is, however, beneficial to apply a magnesium compress to such injuries to speed up the healing process 2 (or more) days later. It will improve blood circulation, help to clear bruises and limit the formation of scar tissue in the area (normally experienced as knots). Whether to use magnesium or not depends very much on the state of an injury and medical advice.

In cases of inflammation (caused, for example, by rheumatoid arthritis) a body temperature magnesium compress may reduce inflammation and pain. If the cause of pain is a chronic condition where inflammation is not present a warm compress is more beneficial. It also works very well on areas where knots have been formed after an injury, as well as in areas of muscle tension, joint pain and other chronic conditions (such as the frozen shoulder, tennis elbow, runner's knee, carpal tunnel syndrome, etc).

How to make a compress

1. You will need a soft absorbent cloth (gauze is good, but other soft absorbent material will be ok too), a bowl with water - hot or cold, magnesium flakes or oil (oil is more expensive than flakes), clingfilm, and a piece of material to hold the compress in place (a wide elastic bandage works well, but so does anything else you can find - even a scarf).
2. For magnesium flakes or Epsom salt - prepare a 1:4 salt to water solution. This will work out as 20g (1 heaped tablespoon) of salt to 80ml (1/6 of a pint) of water, or 40g of salt to 160ml (about 1/3 of a pint) of water.
3. For magnesium oil - add 1 part of magnesium oil to 2 part of water.
4. Soak the cloth in the solution, squeeze excess water out of it.
5. Apply to the area.

6. Wrap with cling film.

7. Wrap with a piece of dry cloth or an elastic bandage.

8. Leave on for 2 hours.

9. For chronic, dull pain a compress can be left on for longer - 3-4 hours, and sometimes even overnight.

10.   If an area treated is inflamed, avoid using hot compresses - body temperature is all that is needed. But before you start any treatment on an inflamed area, seek medical advice.

A compress can be applied as often as necessary, even several times a day - depending on the condition.

Module 19 - Application Methods of Transdermal Magnesium Therapy (Part 2)

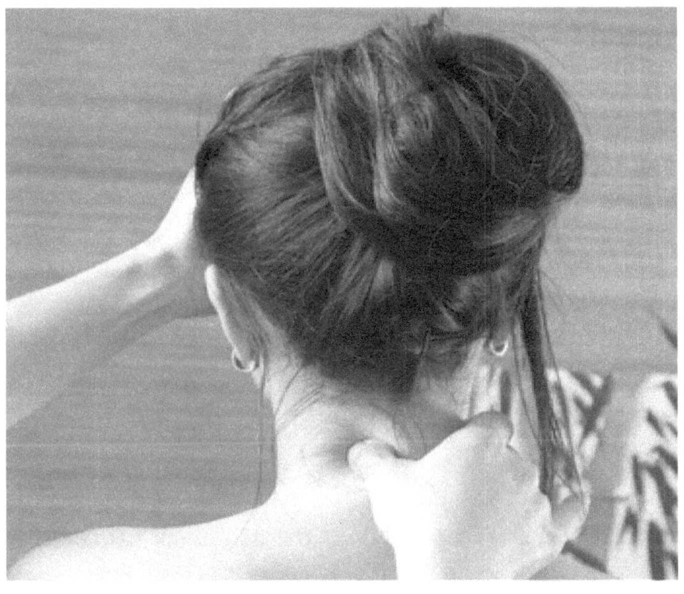

Unit 1 - Magnesium Spray and Body Rub

Magnesium can be applied to the body as a spray or rubbed on the body by hand. Magnesium oil, as well as solutions of magnesium sulphate (Epsom salt) and Dead Sea salt, can be used for this purpose.

Magnesium oil is the most common product for such applications. To apply it by hand, simply put a few drops on the palm of a hand and rub on the area you want to treat. Let it dry and simply leave it on the body to do its work. It can be washed off after about an hour if you feel itchy and uncomfortable. Otherwise, leave it on for the night. To relieve itchiness, add some water to magnesium oil - this will make it less concentrated.

How much and how often?

It depends on your requirements and what you are using it for. If you want to supplement magnesium, spray or rub a magnesium salt solution over the body every day for the first week, every other day for 3 weeks after, and twice a week after that. To treat a condition (e.g. stiffness, pain) use it as often as needed.

Which parts of the body can magnesium salts be used on?

There is no limitation as on which parts of the body magnesium salts can be used since the whole body benefits from it. The only thing is to consider is a personal reaction to it. Some people have dry or very sensitive skin which can get itchy and irritated. While it is not dangerous, it can be unpleasant. In this case, use a less concentrated solution by adding water to it. It also helps to moisturise the skin before application. One of the best moisturiser recipes is warm water followed by an application of coconut oil.

Unit 2 - Far Infrared Magnesium Wrap

Far Infrared (FIR) Magnesium Pain & Health Management Wrap offers a fast-acting solution to back pain, aching muscles and joints, as well as problems connected with magnesium deficiency. The treatment is performed using a far-infrared thermal bag/sauna and magnesium oil, or another magnesium-based product.

The infrared heat penetrates the body tissues promoting their relaxation and speeding up blood circulation, lymph drainage and metabolism. The heat also increases the product interaction with the body and its effect many times. The body tissues relax and pores open up to take in the vital minerals from the products while sweating out the toxins, and aches and pains with them.

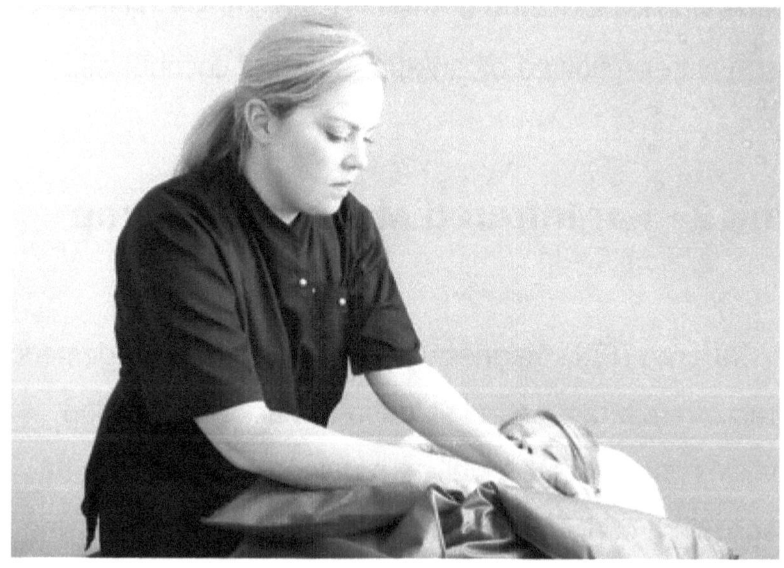

The treatment consists of massage, followed by an application of a magnesium product, after which the client is wrapped in a plastic sheet and placed in the warmed-up infrared thermal sauna bag for 45 minutes (zipped or unzipped – as you prefer). The variation of treatment can be used to soften the strong effects of magnesium salt and far-infrared heat, and prolong the treatment.

Benefits

- Increased circulation
- Remineralisation of the body
- Detoxification of the whole body through profuse sweating and the use of special detoxifying minerals
- Reduction in aches and pains
- Increased energy levels
- Improved sleep
- Skin regeneration
- Reduced puffiness
- Promotion of weight loss
- Relaxation of the body and mind
- Reduction in back tension
- Improved immunity
- Feeling lighter, younger, relaxed and energised.

Contraindications

Not everybody should use the treatment, since there are contraindications to it, such as acute heart conditions, tumours, infections, inflammations, pregnancy, menstruation, undiagnosed lumps, thrombosis, epilepsy, being under the effect of alcohol and drugs among others. If in doubt, consult your GP. It is up to you to make sure that you are in a fit condition to undergo the treatment.

We teach how to do Far Infrared Magnesium Wrap in a separate course - http://courses.purenaturecures.com/fir-magnesium-pain-health-management-wrap/

Unit 3 - Other Applications

Magnesium products can be used in quite a few other ways. Here are some of them:

1. Deodorant - apply magnesium oil under the arms to keep armpits odourless.

2. Acne - mix magnesium oil with water 1:1, apply on the face using hands or cotton wool pads.

3. Natural antibacterial gargle - 1 tbsp of magnesium flakes to 100g of warm water.

4. Sitz bath - 200g of magnesium chloride flakes to 10 litres of warm water to promote a healthy genito-urinary system.

5. Headache rub - rub into the scalp, forehead, on the back of the head and neck to relieve a tension headache.

6. Body scrub - mix magnesium sulphate (Epsom salt) with coconut oil, use as a body scrub to get rid of dead skin.

7. Facial exfoliator - grind magnesium flakes finely, mix with coconut oil or shea butter. Use once a week to exfoliate dead skin.

8. Face mask - mix magnesium oil with water (1:1 or whatever dilution suits your skin type), add to clay or other mask product of your choice for a relaxing and rejuvenating face mask.

Module 20 - Transdermal Magnesium Therapy - Contraindications and Cautions

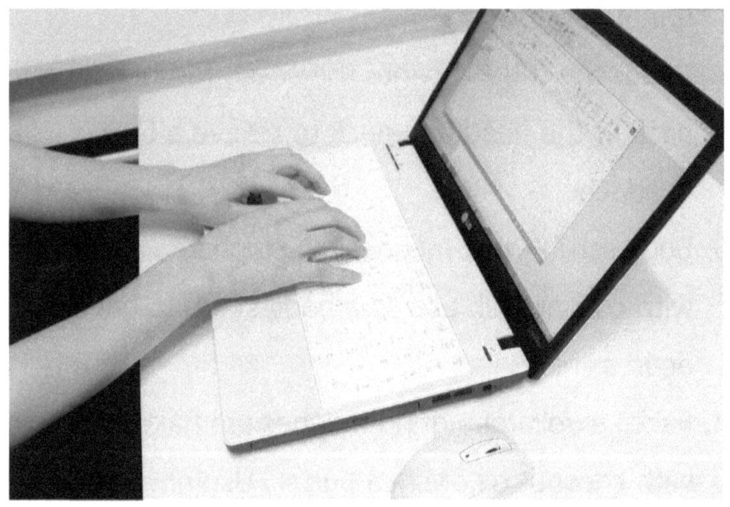

Unit 1 - Contraindications and Cautions

Transdermal Magnesium Therapy (TMT) is safe for most people - safer than with other types of magnesium supplementation. Magnesium toxicity occurs in rare cases, and mostly when too much magnesium has been administered too quickly - intravenously or orally.

However, despite TMT being the safest way to supplement magnesium, in some cases, it may be inappropriate, and caution needs to be exercised. Such cases include, but are not limited to:

- Kidney disorders (people with impaired kidney function may have trouble taking excess magnesium out of the body)
- Low blood pressure (people whose blood pressure is low may have it drop even further after magnesium supplementation)
- People taking blood pressure medication (to exclude interference with magnesium)
- Pregnancy - even though most pregnant women benefit greatly from extra magnesium, it's safest to consult with your GP
- Dehydration due to diarrhoea or excessive sweating (other minerals need to be considered too - such as

calcium, potassium and sodium - to restore the mineral balance)

- Hypothyroidism
- People using magnesium-containing medicines (antacids, laxatives)
- Colitis and gastroenteritis
- Addison's disease
- Sensitive skin (caution - magnesium oil may irritate very sensitive skin, so it is best to dilute magnesium oil with water in the 1:1 ratio).

Symptoms of magnesium toxicity include

- Mental lethargy
- A sudden drop in blood pressure
- Difficulty breathing
- Irregular heartbeat
- Muscle weakness
- Nausea
- Diarrhoea
- Loss of appetite
- Depression.

Magnesium toxicity is a rare condition which is usually caused either by ingesting too much magnesium in one intake intravenously or inability of the body to metabolise it due to kidney problems. The skin protects the body from excessive salt intake, so transdermal magnesium therapy is considered safe. Still, there are certain contra-indications and cautions as mentioned above which need to be observed.

In clinics, magnesium toxicity is offset by injecting calcium chloride intravenously. If you suspect magnesium toxicity, seek medical help immediately - do not resort to self-diagnosis or self-treatment.

The best thing, like with anything new, is to start slowly and observe how the body responds, building up gradually. It is also important to ensure that mineral balance is maintained at all times. Even though magnesium is one of the most important minerals in the body, there are other minerals too which need to be in balance to ensure optimal health.

242

Module 21 - How to Keep Magnesium Level High at All Times

Unit 1 - Magnesium Rich Food & Supplements

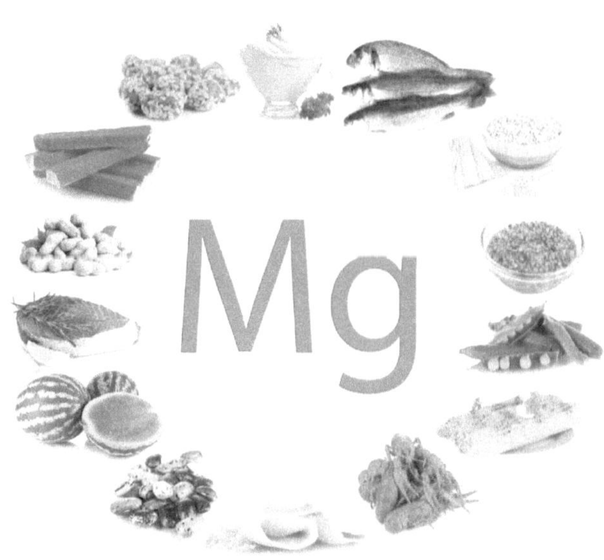

Most of the magnesium we have in our body comes from

food and food supplements. Magnesium-rich food products include:

- Dark leafy greens (spinach, kale)
- Wild (not farmed) fish and seafood
- Nuts (brazil nuts, almonds, peanuts, walnuts)
- Dried fruit (dates, figs, apricots)
- Black-eyed beans
- Pumpkin, sunflower and other seeds
- Yoghurt
- Whole grains
- Dark chocolate
- Bananas
- Avocados
- Broccoli
- Crustaceans
- Watermelons
- Yellow corn
- Dry roasted soybeans
- Coriander
- Artichokes
- Whole milk.

The best magnesium sources are either of organic origin or salts since magnesium from such sources is easily absorbed by the body and doesn't need to drain the body's resources. Magnesium-rich supplements include:

- Spirulina
- Chlorella
- Magnesium Orotate
- Magnesium citrate
- Magnesium Malate
- Magnesium glycinate
- Magnesium carbonate
- Magnesium chloride
- Magnesium sulphate (Epsom salt).

Supplements to avoid:

- Magnesium oxide
- Magnesium aspartate and glutamate.

Magnesium oxide takes stomach acid to break down, so can interfere with digestion. Glutamic and aspartic acids are part of aspartame and become neurotoxic if unbound to other amino acids.

Unit 2 - Anti-Nutrients & Other Things Which Deplete Magnesium Levels

Magnesium deficiency happens not only because the food we eat doesn't have enough of it, but also because of the consumption of substances called "anti-nutrients" which deplete magnesium levels in the body. Such substances include (but are not limited to):

1. Refined carbohydrates
2. Excessive salt intake
3. Artificial sweeteners, colourings and preservatives
4. Trans-fats
5. Smoked meat and fish
6. Fried food
7. Antibiotics

8. Laxatives

9. Certain medicines (e.g. blood pressure medications and a large number of others)

10. Chemotherapy

11. Hormones & plastics we ingest with food and water

12. Heavy metals from food, water and air

13. Pesticides

14. Other environmental toxins

15. "Soft" tap water

16. Soft drinks

17. Alcohol

18. Tobacco

19. Recreational drugs

20. Convenience food

21. Toiletries & cosmetics (try using natural ones)

22. Electromagnetic radiation.

Other things:

1. Excessive sweating due to exercise, strenuous activity or illness

2. Diarrhoea

3. Stress - chronic and acute.

Even the "good" food we eat is often grown in magnesium-poor soil, so cannot provide the amount of magnesium we need for good health. So supplementation becomes the only choice, and transdermal supplementation is the safest way to maintain optimal magnesium level in the body.

Unit 3 - Which Type of Magnesium Is Best?

With so many supplements on the market and ways to supplement magnesium, people often ask themselves a question: shall I take oral supplements or use bath salts? Which supplement is best? Which salt shall I use for baths and other skin applications?

It is impossible to give the answer which suits everyone, for a simple reason that everyone's situation is different. So we can take a look at various forms of magnesium, and a decision will have to be taken in each particular case based on individual circumstances.

Oral magnesium supplements

1. Magnesium oxide is a poorly absorbed form of magnesium since it needs to be broken down by the body, a function which falls on the stomach acid, adding a strain to the digestive system. It also can cause stool softening.
2. Magnesium chloride and lactate have about 12% of magnesium but are more readily absorbed than other forms.
3. Magnesium sulphate - be careful, as it is easy to overdose on it.
4. Magnesium hydroxide (milk of magnesia) - used as a calming remedy for the stomach and a laxative. Be careful to avoid overdosing.
5. Magnesium carbonate has antacid properties, so is not suitable for everyone.
6. Magnesium glycinate (chelated form) - has a reputation as the most efficient supplement due to

the highest absorption and bioavailability. Ideal for those who aim to correct magnesium deficiency.

7. Magnesium taurate (chelated form) - a combination of magnesium and tauric acid. Has a calming effect on the body and mind.
8. Magnesium threonate (chelated) - new supplement which has a higher ability to penetrate the mitochondrial membrane, so is seen as promising.
9. Magnesium citrate (chelated) - a combination of magnesium and citric acid. Has laxative properties.

Transdermal supplementation - which salt is best?

Transdermal supplementation normally uses 2 salts - magnesium chloride and magnesium sulphate. Sometimes Dead Sea salt is used too.

As to which magnesium salt is best, Dr Mark Sircus has the following answer: "According to Daniel Reid, author of The Tao of Detox, magnesium sulfate, commonly known as Epsom salts, is rapidly excreted through the kidneys and therefore difficult to assimilate. This would explain in part why the effects of Epsom salt baths do not last long and why you need more magnesium sulfate in a bath than magnesium chloride to get similar results.

Magnesium chloride is easily assimilated and metabolized in the human body.[1] However, Epsom salts are used specifically by parents of children with autism because of the sulfate, which they are usually deficient in, sulfate is also crucial to the body and is wasted in the urine of autistic children.

For purposes of cellular detoxification and tissue purification, the most effective form of magnesium is magnesium chloride, which has a strong excretory effect on toxins and stagnant energies stuck in the tissues of the body, drawing them out through the pores of the skin. This is a powerful hydrotherapy that draws toxins from the tissues, replenishes the "vital fluid" of the cells and restores cellular magnesium to optimum levels.

Magnesium Chloride is environmentally safe and is used around vegetation and in agriculture. It is not irritating to the skin at lower concentrations and is less toxic than common table salt.

Magnesium Chloride solution was not only harmless for tissues, but it had also a great effect on leucocytic activity and phagocytosis; so it was perfect for external wounds treatment." http://magnesiumforlife.com/product-information/magnesium-chloride-vs-magnesium-sulfate/

Some benefits of transdermal supplementation

1. Magnesium from salts gets absorbed by the body fast, so beneficial effects are felt fast too, by the whole body.
2. There is no risk of overdosing since the skin simply won't absorb more than the body can take.
3. The digestive system does not get involved in breaking down the salts - they get broken down by the water and get into the body in an ionic form.

4. Apart from pain relief, transdermal supplementation offers a whole range of other benefits mentioned in this course.

Module 22 - Therapist Qualification, Additional Information and Further Reading

Unit 1 - Therapist Qualification Requirements

The courses run by the Pure Nature Cures School of Mineral & Spa Therapies are aimed both at therapists and members of the public.

1. Members of the public take our courses to learn about the health benefits of salts, clays and minerals and do treatments on themselves, at their own risk. In the case of existing health issues, members of the public should always seek medical advice before performing any treatment. Even though the predominant majority of people will benefit from the treatments to some they may be contra-indicated or performed with caution.

2. Our courses can also be taken by qualified massage and beauty therapists who would like to add new skills to their portfolio. To be deemed qualified, a therapist needs to have a Level 3 Anatomy & Physiology and Body Massage Diploma.

3. While all the students will be issued with the Certificate of Completion, only qualified therapists will receive a certificate which will give them an opportunity to apply for Practitioner insurance and treat members of the public.

4. We cannot guarantee that the qualification we offer will be accepted by insurers in the countries outside

the EU, due to variations regarding requirements for complementary therapies. Please enquire with your local insurance providers.

5. To qualify as a therapist, you will need to sign up for the add-on short course for therapists which covers subjects such as hygiene, professional issues and case studies.

6. The practical one-day module is offered to therapists in the UK & Northern Ireland, as well as to those who can travel to the UK for the course.

Unit 2 – Additional Reading

1.   Transdermal Magnesium Therapy, Dr Mark Sircus.

2.   The Miracle of Magnesium, Carolyn Dean, M.D., N.D.

3.   Magnesium in Clinical practice, J Durlach.

4.   Magnesium Deficiency in the Pathogenesis of Disease, Early Roots of Cardiovascular, Skeletal, and Renal Abnormalities, Seelig M S.

5.	http://www.magnesiumeducation.com

6.	http://www.mgwater.com/

7.	Magnesium Requirements in Human Nutrition, Seelig M S.

8.	_The requirement of magnesium by the normal adult,_ Seelig M S.

9.	The high heart health value of drinking-water magnesium, Andrea Rosanoff.

10.	Magnesium homeostasis and aging, Mario Barbagallo, Mario Belvedere, Ligia J. Dominguez

11.	Sheehan JP, Seelig MS: _Magnesium, potassium and arrhythmias._

Further Information

Did you find information in this book useful? Leave feedback to me know what you think! Would you like to learn more? I have published a number of books on the subject of minerals. You can find them on Amazon.

Mineral Healing Books

1. **Earth's Humble Healers:** Learn How to Use Salts, Muds & Clays for Better Health, Youth & Vitality. Plus 80 Health & Beauty Recipes

2. **How Clays Work:** Science & Applications of Clays & Clay-like Minerals in Health & Beauty

3. **Magnesium at Home:** 25 Most Common Health Conditions & How Magnesium Salts Can Help

4. **Mineral Healing Recipe Book:** An overview of how minerals can be used in everyday life to address common health problems, boost health and vitality.

5. **Introduction to Mineral Healing**
Learn interesting facts about healing properties of salts, muds, clays, zeolite and diatomaceous earth. It is a good

Transdermal Magnesium Therapy Course for Clinic & Home Use

book to start learning about minerals.

6. **<u>First Aid Guide to Minerals</u>**

Find out how salts, muds and clays can help when medicines are unavailable.

Courses

1. **Far Infrared Mineral Weight Loss Wrap Course** for Clinic & Home Use: Learn how to use clays, salts and far infrared for sustainable weight loss and better health

https://www.amazon.com/dp/B07N99H1XV

2. **Far Infrared Magnesium Wrap Course for Clinic & Home Use**: Learn how to use magnesium salts and far infrared for better health and vitality

https://www.amazon.com/dp/B07JZDWQX1

3. **Transdermal Magnesium Therapy Course for Clinic & Home Use**

https://www.amazon.com/dp/B07GXXGWT7

4. **Far Infrared Clay Detox Wrap Course for Clinic & Home Use:** Learn how to use clays and far infrared for transdermal detox and healing

https://www.amazon.com/dp/B07JCL55TZ

5. **Forever Young: Far Infrared Remineralising & Rejuvenating Seaweed Wrap Course**: Learn how to use the power of the sun, the earth & the ocean to stay young, vibrant and healthy

https://www.amazon.com/dp/B097CWDCG4

If you prefer to read books in the **PDF format**, you can buy them here:

https://purenaturecures.com/book-shop

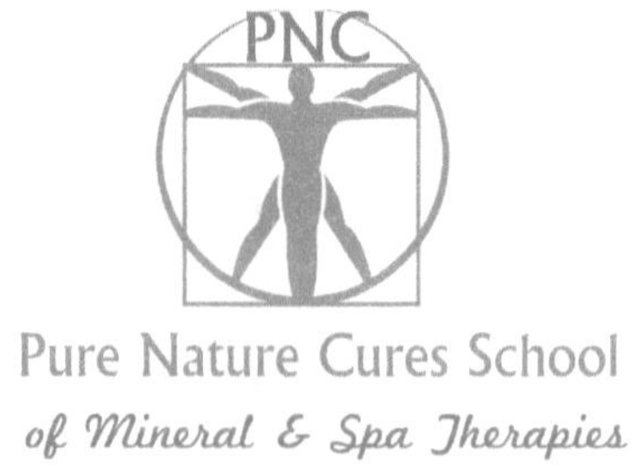

Pure Nature Cures School
of Mineral & Spa Therapies